'thin secrets'

how to be slim without dieting

Lizzie Kingsley PhD

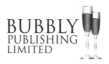

BUBBLY
PUBLISHING
LIMITED

Thin Secrets: How to be slim without dieting
Lizzie Kingsley Ph.D.

First published in Great Britain in December 2006 by Bubbly Publishing Limited, P.O. Box 4127 Sheffield, S10 9BP.

ISBN 10: 0-9554111-0-6
ISBN 13: 978-0-9554111-0-6

Printed in the UK by The Alden Press, Oxford

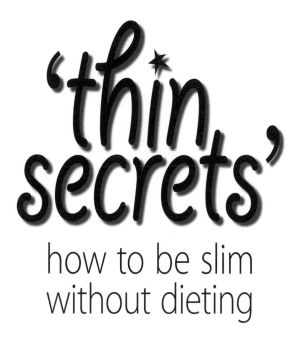

'thin secrets'

how to be slim
without dieting

Lizzie Kingsley PhD

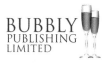

BUBBLY
PUBLISHING
LIMITED

Acknowledgements

Many, many people have helped with the research into *Thin Secrets*. In particular I would like to thank 'the family' – mum and dad, Sarah, Cathal, Annie and Catherine; Mel, Binns, Nikki and Tim. Thanks for the support and feedback. I am grateful that I have been able to mention some of you when recounting my journey to slimness. Thanks also go to my case studies for letting me use their stories – you all know who you are.

In addition, I have received a great amount of help and encouragement from Dorothy Trump, Jo Smith, Rosie Burgess, Helen Spencer and Midori Kayahara.

I would also like to acknowledge and thank Kate Timmins for copyediting, as well as Anna, Lucy and the team at Carnegie who turned the manuscript into a proper book.

Last, but most certainly not least, I would like to thank my husband James who has read and re-read countless drafts of this book. As a genuine follower of the 'living slim' philosophy, his honest and constructive feedback has been priceless. I dedicate this book to him.

Contents

Preface
Hollow legs?

Many, many years ago, around about the time that I believed in Santa Claus and the Tooth Fairy, I was told that I had hollow legs. I took this 'fact' at face value, for a while – truly believing that my legs must be empty – before I began to question the wisdom of the older generation! Long before the Tooth Fairy paid her final visit, I learnt that my legs were no different from anybody else's; however the idea that I could eat anything I wanted to, and not gain any weight, had already been passed on to me. I had been singled out as being a bit different to others – including my three sisters – and it's only now, twenty years on, that I am beginning to realise the impact that this has had.

Obviously, nobody has hollow legs. I have no idea where the expression originated from, or how long ago it was first used; however, it shows that the observation that some people seem to be able to 'get away with it' has been around for a while. How can one person appear to have a huge appetite and remain slim, whereas another person may eat the same amount, or even less, and still have a weight problem?

This little issue has bugged many of us at some time or another, and most of us have probably reasoned that there must be something different about these slim people. Okay, its not that they have any extra storage room in their legs, but they must be just naturally thinner, right? Well that's what I always thought, until recently that is.

I admit, I was always quite skinny throughout my school years. It seemed perfectly reasonable to me at the time, that some people were just naturally slimmer than others, in the same way that some people are naturally taller than all of their peers. I was so used to being a 'naturally' slim person by the time I went to university, I felt that I could almost eat whatever I pleased and not suffer the consequences of weight gain in the same way as everybody else seemed to.

For a while it seemed to work. Eventually though, I began to gain weight – only gradually and steadily – however my normal weight became a few pounds more than it had been previously. Fortunately, I would lose some of the weight that I had gained each term, during the university vacations. So I finished my three years a little bit heavier than I began, but I reasoned that so did everyone else!

Meanwhile, I began to notice that some of the people around me, who had also been gaining weight, had gone from carrying around a couple of extra pounds, to the beginnings of having real weight issues. Over the next few years a gap began to emerge between two sets of people. There were the 'naturally' slim people on one side of the gap; these were the people that had never had a weight problem and therefore had also never been on a diet. On the other side were the people that continued to put on weight, regardless of whether they dieted or not, until one day they realised that the few pounds had turned into stones.

I was in the middle of this somewhere. Up until that point I had always been on the slim side of the gap (albeit gaining weight at a steady rate). Although I had put weight on, I didn't do anything about it until it started to affect my dress size. At that point, I tried dieting, but usually only managed a week or two at a time. Even when I dieted successfully and lost a few pounds, I would regain it again fairly quickly once I came off the diet and the overall trend of gaining weight would continue.

I quickly became fed up with yo-yo dieting and never seeming to really make progress, so I began to change my approach to weight control. Over time, my weight seemed to stabilise. I stopped gaining weight and gradually I started to lose it again. The more weight I lost, the more effort I put into 'becoming slim', using the new approach that I had learnt.

I didn't really realise the significance of any of this until I was chatting to my sister over dinner one day. She made a throwaway comment about me being naturally slim, bringing back memories of my 'hollow legs' days. That was when it struck me, that these two groups of people, the 'naturally' slim and the less fortunate, were not fundamentally different. If I was still perceived as being naturally slim, when I actively had to control my weight, then maybe it was the same for everyone else who I had previously thought of as naturally thin. I realised that, in my adult years, I was not naturally slim, and I had had to make a choice. Once I had lost weight, I did not want to gain too much again, and so I had begun to put real effort into staying slim. At the same time, the people around me assumed that it came quite naturally to me. Were all the other slim people working just as hard?

That would mean that the slim people had not been dealt a better hand genetically, they had just been instinctively more aware of the rules of the game. Others, who didn't feel in control of their weight, were only at a disadvantage because they didn't know the secrets of staying slim.

I was told as a child that I was a slim person – that I was lucky. Being slim brought me a fair bit of (mostly) positive attention. When I began to put weight on, I lost some of that. This may have been a motivator for me to turn the trend from steadily gaining weight to slimming down again. In a way, as a child I was handed a self-fulfilling prophecy, which has resulted in me putting effort into remaining slim, but at the same time feeling like I had a little bit of a natural advantage.

If that was really the case for me, were there people out there who had been given the idea that they are more prone to weight gain and there was nothing that they could do about it? Ironically, if they did put on weight, then it would appear to prove the theory in the first place.

Is there any such thing as a 'naturally' slim person?

The idea that some people were just naturally slim was really called into question. What made them naturally slim? Was it that they had inherited good genes that meant that they could eat whatever they pleased and do very little exercise without putting on any weight? Did that mean that there were people who believed that they were naturally overweight and, regardless of what they did, they would never be slim?

The idea fascinated me and I began to observe other people's behaviour and their attitudes. I also wondered whether there were real physical, or biological, explanations that could account for why some people gained weight whilst others remained slim for life. At the time I was researching for my doctorate in Medical Genetics, and thought that some of the published research in my chosen field could possibly provide me with the answers. Maybe there was a genetic reason why some people stayed slim and others were more prone to weight gain?

Although I found that there were several, quite serious, inherited genetic disorders which caused weight gain in a very small number of people, it seemed that 'genetics' could not explain the difference between the people who gained too much weight and the others who remained slim. Meanwhile, I also found out that it was not just me that had been raised with the belief that some people were just born lucky, and others were not. The majority of people that I talked to on the subject also believed that a large element of luck was involved. In the course of researching *Thin Secrets* I carried out a survey on people's attitude to their weight. To my surprise, 95% of the respondents reported that they believed that some people were naturally thin.

The more I learnt about the differences between people who

remained slim and those that did not, the more I realised that there were certain attitudes and behaviours that were different between the two groups. These two sets of people are not separated by a genetic luck-of-the-draw, or any natural advantage, but the slim people behaved in different ways. Moreover, these 'slim' ways can be learnt! I was left with a dilemma, do I go with the flow and carry on as a 'lucky' person, or was it time to start sharing the secrets to losing weight and staying slim for life?

I began to realise that these misconceptions were possibly holding some people back in their attempts at weight loss. If they truly believed that they were not a naturally slim person, how then could they ever hope to achieve a slim figure? More interestingly, I started to think that maybe the expectation for a slim child or teenager to stay slim into their adult years might, ironically, provide the motivation for them to stay slim (as it did in my case). This was not a difference of biology, or genetics; this was all about expectations.

The key to successful permanent weight loss lies in attitude. The *Thin Secrets* that we will uncover in this book, all show how the attitudes that slim people have help them to remain slim. Slim people know the *Thin Secrets* and that is their advantage. You too can learn the *Thin Secrets*. Up until now, all the strategies for weight loss have put far too much emphasis on what the overweight person is doing 'wrong' – I believe that focusing on what the slim person is doing 'right' is the key to successful, permanent weight loss.

The advantage of the *Thin Secrets* is that just understanding and accepting them can dramatically improve your chances of successful weight loss. If what you learn in this book changes your attitude to your weight, then a natural change in your behaviour will follow. In future, losing weight will not be a miserable process with the feeling of deprivation that can accompany a diet. Instead you will have the confidence to become a slim person and enjoy the process.

This book will challenge the idea that there is a natural advantage when it comes to being slim. It is all down to certain attitudes and behaviours which can be learnt. Anybody can achieve it. Hopefully, what we uncover in this book will lead to more successful long-term weight loss than could be achieved by dieting. By 'thinking slim', you will feel more in control of your weight and at the same time ensure that you will never again have to diet. Imagine that,

No more diets!

'Thin Secrets'

What can we learn from slim people?

Everybody knows a 'naturally' slim person. They are the sort of person who can get away with eating whatever they please. They never diet – they don't need to because they are slim.

Maybe you have a friend who you occasionally meet for dinner. Years ago, you were both slim, now it's just her. Yet she can eat her way through three courses with gusto, and polish off enough wine to keep the Catholic church going until Christmas! How did she manage to stay slim over the years when you didn't? How can she possibly eat so much and get away with it? Is she just lucky? Or is she naturally slim?

Maybe you work with someone who has never had a weight problem? When the cakes or biscuits are being passed around at coffee-time, there is no fuss from her. Whereas the rest of the room are exchanging the customary "ooh, I really shouldn't", and "the diet can start tomorrow" comments, the annoyingly slim person just eats and enjoys.

What can we learn from these people? Are there rules that we can apply to our own lives, which will guarantee slimness for life? How come dieting gets us nowhere? What are the *Thin Secrets?*

I decided to write this book to share some of the secrets. These are not guidelines about what to eat, or when to eat. The secrets are how slim people manage to maintain their figures seemingly effortlessly. In fact, the secrets are actually what many slim people know and do instinctively. As a result, they can be so ingrained that many slim people are not actually aware of them.

The others, who know the secrets, may not want you to find out. It will take away from their mystery. They will no longer be someone who 'has it all' and they will just be a normal person who knows what it is they have to do to remain slim.

On top of all this, the diet industry thrives on you buying in to the next miracle fad diet. They don't want you to 'go it alone'. Where would the diet industry be if everyone lost weight and stayed slim for life?

I discovered the secrets by observing different types of people and talking to them about their attitudes and their habits. I also find that knowing the *Thin Secrets* has helped enormously with my own personal weight control. If you apply the *Thin Secrets*, you will be able to relax about your weight. Your ideal body weight will become achievable, not by dieting, but by living like a slim person. Eventually, you will also learn how to enjoy food without feeling guilty. No foods are banned when you live like a slim person.

Knowing the *Thin Secrets* should help both people who are trying to lose weight and those, who are already slim, who want to understand how to stay slim for the rest of their lives. Although everyone can use the *Thin Secrets*, throughout the book I often assume that the reader is interested in losing weight. I apologise if this does not apply to you, but I hope that you will still gain a lot from this book. Understanding all the *Thin Secrets* will make it easier for you to maintain your slim figure, just as it has helped me.

This is no miracle cure for excess weight – nor is it a fad diet. This is about changing your attitude to weight control which should ensure a steady and healthy rate of weight loss. The *Thin Secrets* will help anybody who has the goal of maintaining a slim figure – permanently. You are totally in control and able to determine your own rate of progress – after all, it's your life we are talking about.

In the first section of the book I will describe the nine *Thin Secrets*. The advantage with most of these is that just knowing them will change your attitude to your weight. This will, in turn, help to change your approach to weight loss. However, some secrets require a little more understanding and practice before they can be applied to maximum effect to help you to lose weight.

The second part of the book will build on the *Thin Secrets*, allowing you to see for yourself how having a 'slim' approach to your weight can be successful. The book progresses from how to 'Think slim', to how to 'Act Slim' and finally on to how to 'Be slim'. Although it is the later part of the book which focuses on a weight-loss strategy it is important to read all the way through to get to grips with slim thinking before trying to put it into practice.

Hopefully, by the time you have finished reading this book you will be thinking like a slim person, allowing you to begin to act like a slim person, which is the ultimate key to actually becoming one.

A word of warning before we begin though – the inspiration for this book came from being told that I was 'naturally' thin. The idea that some people have a natural advantage has often been used as an easy way to explain why some people are slim, seemingly without effort. I intend to challenge this assumption, so I am asking you to keep an open mind during the first section of the book. Many people have immediately rejected the first of the *Thin Secrets* when it was presented to them. This is because the idea had never been challenged before. It is necessary, in order to be able to think like a slim person, to try to understand all of the *Thin Secrets*. Stick with it and all will be explained ...

SOMETHING

There is no such thing as a
ordinary salesperson

Secret One

"There is no such thing as a 'naturally' slim person"

Many slim people think that there is a certain element of luck in being slim, in the same way that overweight people may think that they are less lucky. Luck definitely plays a part, but not in the way that you might expect. The big secret is that slim people are not 'genetically' lucky. They were not born with it and neither are they 'naturally' slim. However, they have had the good fortune to have learnt attitudes and habits (usually from a young age) which have kept them slim. All these people have to do to stay slim for life is to carry on behaving exactly as they always have done.

The reason that they, and everyone else, think that they are naturally slim, is because they are so used to thinking and acting like a slim person, it just appears to come naturally to them. Put it this way, if these 'naturally' slim people binged on all of the 'wrong' foods and didn't do any exercise, they would eventually get fat! In my lifetime, I do not think that I have met one truly naturally slim person – someone who can eat lots of high-fat foods, do no exercise and still not put weight on.

I have, however, met lots of people who thought that they were naturally slim, until we started to talk about their attitudes, habits and lifestyle, and identified that they are just very well practised slim people.

Some people do not know what it is that keeps them slim – they wrongly assume that it is 'genetic' luck

These slim people behave in different ways to those who tend to put weight on. As these differences can be quite subtle they are often not easy to spot. More importantly, these 'lucky' people actually have very different attitudes to food and to being slim – and that is NOT BECAUSE they are slim, it is WHY they are slim. This means that there is the potential for anybody to learn how to be slim.

To clarify, the slim people that I talk about in this book are everyday people who maintain a healthy weight. They are people that you know, who live life to the full, and stay slim. I would not encourage anybody to aim to be very thin, or promote the sort of figure that can only arise from an eating disorder – I am also a bit wary about some of our celebrity role models. Our role models should be those real people who are healthily slim, who maintain that slimness without resorting to drastic measures, or playing dangerous games with their health.

Okay, there are some people who seem blessed with a very nice body shape. You know the ones who seem to store any excess fat in all the right places first, so will gain a nice curvy figure, rather than carry a few pounds around the middle. These people do gain weight; however, they get away with it for a bit longer than most. They are still looking good, while the rest of us are starting to feel a little flabby. There are others who may appear to gain weight at a much slower rate then most. Everyone is slightly different; however, MOST people that we view as naturally slim have in fact LEARNT how to be slim.

Is body weight genetic?

Many people, both those who are overweight and those who are slim, believe that their body weight is genetic. They think that they are generally stuck with what they have got, because that is what they inherited. Although our genes are partly responsible for our body weight and shape, it is very unlikely that the weight that you are at the moment is genetic. This is because how we live our lives, how much we eat, or don't eat, and how much we exercise has a huge impact on our weight. The effect of our lifestyle or 'environment' on our weight is so large that it can outdo the small part played by genetics.

As an example, consider identical twins. They are completely genetically identical. Let us assume that they have very similar body weights to start with. If one twin ate more than they needed to, and didn't do any exercise, whereas the other twin had a very healthy diet and did plenty of exercise, then quite soon there would be a very big difference in weight between the two of them. Their genetics are still identical, but it is their environments that are having the biggest impact on their weights.

Incidentally, we often find that identical twins have similar weights to each other, as they have very similar habits and lifestyles. So although it would appear that their weight is purely genetic, it is in fact their similar environments that are playing a big role in keeping their weights comparable.

It is easy to think that just because our parents or our siblings are overweight that it is a family thing. In the same way, there are many families where everyone is slim. It just seems to follow that it is genetic, but that is only part of the story. Anyone can be slim, regardless of whether the rest of their family is overweight. If your environment is slim, you will be too.

Slim people are not genetically slim, but have avoided gaining weight by carefully controlling their environment. Luckily you can learn how to do this to lose weight and stay slim for life.

Most people know what to do to lose weight, but how do we become slim for the rest of our lives?

What about 'natural' body shape?

Everybody has the potential to be slim, but this is not to say that we can all have a figure like Catherine Zeta-Jones, or Angelina Jolie. Your body shape is largely inherited, although it can vary depending on your weight. However, it is unlikely that it will completely change just because you have lost a few pounds... or stones! If you have a small chest relative to your hips, then this probably won't change very much, even if you reduce your body size. If this is the case your hips are likely to always be bigger in proportion to your bust, but you can still achieve slim hips. Obviously, your bone size does not alter, but the amount of fat that you store in that area will, making your hips look considerably slimmer!

Likewise, if you are top-heavy, then it is likely that you will always have a big bust relative to the rest of your body. However, regardless of your body shape, you can still be slim.

Your proportions can change a little bit – I know someone who has a lovely hourglass figure when she is reasonably slim but she tends to gain weight around the middle first, so when she puts weight on, she loses the wonderful waistline. Likewise if she loses a lot of weight then the hips and bust start to slim down as well, reducing the hourglass effect somewhat (but she has to be quite underweight for that to happen, which is not advisable). At the right weight, she has a very enviable figure.

Unless you have previously observed the areas that you tend to put weight on, or lose weight from, then it is difficult to predict how fabulous your figure will be when you do lose weight. You may find that your top-heaviness evens out a lot, or that you become less pear-shaped, when you slim down.

I don't know how many times I have heard the expression "I'm just big-boned". Someone with "bigger bones" may weigh more, but they can still be slim – there will be more about this in a later chapter.

There is also a tendency to think that muscular women can never look very slim. If you build up muscle whilst you are slimming down, you will always look muscular, although you can still be slim. I have always admired the model, Nell McAndrew. She has previously trained very hard for competitive sporting events, such as the London Marathon. This has obviously caused her to build up muscle, but she is still slim and has a very enviable figure. A person with lots of muscle may weigh more than someone else the same size, who has less muscle, but both will be slim. Whatever your body type, you can be slim.

Although your genetics may prevent you from looking like a super-model (unless you are 5'11" with high cheekbones, and a killer pout!), 'genetics' does not prevent you from being slim. When it comes to weight control, there is not a group of people out there that was born lucky. No one has a 'natural' or genetic advantage when it comes to being slim.

The knowledge, that very few people can actually claim to be 'natu-rally' slim, helps us enormously. Firstly, it helps us psychologically. By knowing that the next woman, although she might be slim, does not have any natural advantage, will help reassure us that we can change our weight. It will motivate us to do something about it. Anyone can be slim – YOU can be slim. Secondly, there are masses of people who are all well-practised in the art of 'being slim'. They are all around us and we can learn from them.

So what is different about slim people?

For most people it is hard work to stay slim; it does not just come naturally. This may sound odd, especially as we have just discussed how much it seems to come naturally to them. The point is that it SEEMS to you that being slim doesn't require them to put any effort in; however if you were to look closely at their lifestyle, you would quickly see the ways that they have avoided putting on weight. Slim people are so used to their little habits and attitudes that they may not see them as work, they are just routine. However, if you were to take up all their habits straight away, it would probably feel like work!

Most slim people are very aware of the fact that if they overate, ate the 'wrong' sorts of food, and did very little exercise, then they would get fat. They have decided that they are not going to put weight on, and they make their eating decisions based on this attitude. This will have been done gradually, unlike deciding to go on a diet where you are trying to change all your habits in one day. Instead the slim person has probably spent many years refining all their little habits, until they get to the stage where they have a routine which keeps them slim. As this is a slow process, many people will not be aware that it is even taking place.

Obviously, there are some slim people who exercise a lot and eat healthily. The reasons why they are slim are transparent. These are the people who really deserve their slim toned bodies, as they have put effort into achieving them. Anybody could be this type of slim person too, and everyone knows someone like this. They may cycle to work everyday, and play squash at lunchtimes, while their weekends are spent walking in the hills, or training for a marathon. Often there is no conscious decision to be slim for these people, but the effort goes into being as fit and healthy as possible. They enjoy being fit, and often get a buzz from a competitive sport, or a challenging physical event. A side effect of this very healthy lifestyle is a very healthy weight and a slim body!

In general, we are not jealous of this type of person, as we know that they work at being slim. However, most slim people do not fit into this category. They may not even seem to be particularly healthy, they're just slim. It appears that they eat the same amount that you do, it seems that they don't do very much exercise – why are they slimmer than you are, is it fair?

It would only be unfair if it really was the case that thin people have the same lifestyle that overweight people have. Although they SEEM to have the same lifestyle and not put on weight, it is quite likely that they are very different once you look beyond the small part that you see.

Let's go back to the example of the friend that you regularly meet for dinner – the one that can easily put away three courses. You know that she CAN eat a lot. You know that she DOES eat a lot every once in a while, when she is out with you. Other than the fact that she hasn't gained much weight, do you really know very much about her lifestyle? You may know this person very well, but do you know what she regularly eats for breakfast, or lunch, or whether she has regular snacks? Do you know how often she exercises? Maybe she doesn't have an exercise routine as such, but she has a dog that she takes for a walk twice a day.

Likewise, the slim person at work who always eats the treats at coffee-time – why is she not fat? Do you know whether she eats three meals a day, or whether she eats very small meals several times a day? Maybe, by coffee-time, she is very hungry after her early morning run! The point is that we often only see a small part of the bigger picture.

In order to understand why someone is slim, we have to look at their whole lifestyle. Often we can make very broad generalisations about someone from only seeing a snapshot of the whole. Do not automatically assume that a slim person, who eats something 'naughty', is just lucky to not put weight on. They may only do that occasionally, but because you see it regularly, you assume that it is indicative of their whole lifestyle. They may not eat any other high fat food for the rest of the week.

Instead of just assuming that they are lucky, start thinking about that person as someone who has managed to achieve a terrific balance, and learn from them. They can eat the occasional treat and have the occasional indulgence, without feeling guilty AND without putting on weight. This is not because they were born with a natural advantage of always being slimmer than you. It is because they make up for it in other areas of their lifestyle.

Just because somebody <u>can</u> eat a lot, it doesn't mean that they <u>usually</u> do

A slim person who has a nice balance in their lifestyle can avoid putting on weight. They often make 'slim' choices as part of their normal lifestyle. These may be choices that you would associate with dieting; however, slim people do not starve themselves, or skip meals, or feel deprived. I am talking about everyday decisions being taken with staying slim in mind, such as opting for a jacket potato instead of chips, passing on the cooked breakfast and having cereal, or not having desserts regularly (these are just examples, they are not the ultimate 'rules' for being slim). If slim choices are a major part of your normal lifestyle, then there is no need to feel guilty about the odd 'non-slim' choice. If the slim lifestyle is disrupted a bit, by indulging, or overeating, it is easy to bring it back into balance again quickly.

The slim person who overdoes it a bit at the weekend, is likely to cut back a bit during the week to compensate. By 'compensate' I do not mean crash diet. Instead, they may be a bit more careful with their food choices, or do a bit more exercise for a few days to make up for the binge at the weekend. As these slim people are very well practised at being slim, this compensation is normal to them, and therefore does not feel like a hardship, or a diet.

Lisa

Lisa lived a slim lifestyle. During the week she would usually go for a run on two or three separate occasions, and also tried to fit in a circuit training or aerobics class. Her diet consisted of cereal for breakfast, a packed-lunch of home-made sandwiches, and on most days she would cook a healthy, balanced dinner for herself. She generally didn't snack on chocolate, biscuits or crisps. However, most weekends, Lisa would rest from exercise and would go to visit friends, or family. Obviously, she would eat whatever her hosts provided – and she had a big appetite. Lisa's mother in particular liked to try and feed her up, and she could not understand how her daughter could eat so much food and still not gain any weight.

I am sure that the people who only saw Lisa at the weekend thought she was a 'naturally' slim person! However, if Lisa lived her weekend lifestyle all week, she would very quickly gain weight. Lisa's normal lifestyle during the week compensated for her weekends and acted to regulate her weight.

To outsiders, this may seem like a lot of work. It may even seem to be almost as hard as dieting. Dieting, by its very nature involves restricting yourself to either smaller portions, or to certain types of food. Slim people do not feel restricted, as the compensation is part of their normal lifestyle. It does not require them to go hungry, or to ban carbs, or only eat lettuce. All they are doing is making an effort to make 'slim' choices, which they are used to doing anyway as part of their normal lifestyle. The compensation periods are very much worth being able to occasionally indulge, not feel guilty and not put weight on. These compensations become habit quite quickly and therefore feel less and less like hard work.

Lisa is an example of the 'normal' type of slim person. They are the ones that we can learn from. These people are very good at 'being slim', they have honed it to perfection. The rest of the *Thin Secrets* all focus on how these people manage to maintain such a good balance. We will find out what sets them apart, and how we can learn from them, lose weight, and stay slim permanently. Don't be put off at this stage if you don't like the idea of running twice a week, the key is to find out what will work for you.

Most slim people compensate for indulgences so that overall they do not gain weight

What about the ones that 'get away with it'?

There is a group of slim people however, who throw a spanner in the works. These are the exceptions; the ones that confuse everyone, as they really do appear to get away with eating whatever they please, whenever they please without putting weight on. They are still not 'naturally' slim, although it really does seem like being slim comes naturally to them. This group needs a little bit of explanation, before we can get on with learning the rest of the *Thin Secrets*.

These are the people who appear to always eat junk food, never do any exercise and yet still do not put on weight. What is their secret, if they are not naturally slim? If they are missing out on the compensation period – which is necessary for most people to remain slim – how come they haven't put weight on?

These are likely to be people who do not know what it is that keeps them slim and they probably just assume that they are born with it. This strengthens the idea that they are just lucky, and in a way they are, as they have managed to stumble across a mechanism that will keep them slim without them really working at it. However, if that mechanism were to change, or to fail, they would find themselves gaining weight and they won't really know why. These people tend to fit into one, or more, of three groups.

Group One

The first set is very simple to explain. They are teenagers and young adults who are still growing. This is especially the case for young men, who may have long ago finished growing height-wise, but who might still be broadening out. Many of these 'lucky' people will find that they put weight on in their twenties if their lifestyle remains the same as it was in their teens. This is because the growth spurt that was acting as their compensation mechanism finishes.

Never compare your weight to that of a teenager – it is not a level playing field!

Group Two

The second set of people who SEEM to get away with eating lots of junk food may not eat as much as you think they do. If they did eat too much fatty and sugary food then they would put weight on. Someone who grazes on sweets all day in the office may not actually have a dinner when they get home from work, as they are not hungry. Alternatively, the slim person that has takeaways every evening may not eat very much during the day, or may not actually have a big portion. It all comes down to energy balance. It is possible to eat all the 'wrong' foods and still not put weight on as long as you are not consuming more energy than you are using up (although this is not very healthy).

Group Three

The third set of people who SEEM to get away with it have tipped the energy balance the other way. These are people who are more active than it first appears, and may be using up more energy than you would predict. This could be due to an active job. A hospital doctor may walk several miles and be standing up for hours on a typical shift, whereas a GP may be sitting in a very comfortable chair for most of the day. After a couple of years, there is likely to be a noticeable effect from these different sorts of work.

Having an active job can easily add to your daily energy expenditure, without feeling like exercise. Other less noticeable forms of exercise can soon add up and have an effect on weight, including lots of walking, gardening, or housework. There are also people who use up a great deal of nervous energy. By this, I mean those people who fidget, or pace the room; the ones that are always drumming their fingers or tapping their foot. It doesn't sound like an awful lot, but all that extra calorie usage added up over the course of the day or week could be quite substantial. This may be a common, hidden mechanism for staying slim.

Slim people are not just lucky to be slim; MOST of them keep a balance in their lifestyle which prevents them from gaining weight. The more they are in the habit of 'living like a slim person' then the more naturally it appears to be for them. Although a minority of slim people appear to defy the rules, there is usually an obvious lifestyle reason which can explain how someone has avoided weight gain. You probably know someone who you assumed was naturally slim. Try and identify what it is that is keeping them slim.

> ## To understand the person who appears to 'get away with it' you must look more closely at their lifestyle

Gary

My friend Jo was very interested in the ideas behind this book. When we got talking about "Secret One" – that there was no such thing as a 'naturally' slim person – she immediately protested using her brother Gary as an example. Gary is tall and slim, never seems to eat healthily and very rarely exercises. Jo was adamant that she had found the example that disproved the theory, so we talked about Gary for a while. It was obvious that he was not controlling his weight with a careful diet, and plenty of exercise. At the age of 30, we can also safely assume that Gary had stopped growing. It took us a while to find the reason, but eventually Jo mentioned that Gary always left some food on his plate at the end of every meal. It wasn't a deliberate attempt to waste food; however, it indicated that he stopped eating when he felt full, ensuring that he did not overeat. Jo also realised that her brother's annoying habit of pacing the room instead of sitting down to watch the television, especially when the football was on, was also contributing to him staying so slim.

Although Gary was not fit and healthy, his habits, including fidgeting a lot and not overeating, had kept him from gaining weight. If he ever started to eat everything on his plate, and regularly sat down to watch television, he would undoubtedly begin to gain weight. Luckily for Gary, there is no need for him to change the habits of a lifetime, and therefore he will probably remain slim for some time yet.

What about metabolic rate?

"What about metabolism?" I hear you cry. Surely having a high metabolic rate is a 'natural' advantage when it comes to being slim? Differences in metabolic rate have often been used to explain why some people seem to eat a lot without putting on any weight and others seem to have trouble keeping excess weight off. There are natural variations in metabolism, but it is often assumed that these account for why some people are slimmer than others.

Your metabolic rate relates to the amount of energy that your body uses up over a period of time – the number of calories that you burn up in a day. Taller people tend to burn up more calories than shorter people because they have bigger bodies which require more energy. Also, metabolic rates tend to decrease as we get older because we lose muscle mass. Although there are variations from person to person, with men having higher rates than women, it is possible to increase or decrease our own metabolic rate by changing our lifestyles. Contrary to popular belief you are not stuck with a 'fast' or 'slow' metabolism for life.

While many people get quite concerned about it, metabolic rate can be a bit of a red herring in weight control. Yes, it is true that taller and younger people tend to need more calories to do exactly the same things as others, but gaining weight can increase your metabolic rate as well. Heavier people burn up more calories than lighter people as their bigger bodies use up more energy. There will be more detail about this later on in the book.

Other factors which can affect metabolism include not eating regularly (skipping breakfast), dieting and not being physically active. These all act to slow our metabolic rate and therefore make it harder to lose weight as our bodies will burn fewer calories per day. On the flip side increasing activity levels and building up more muscle tissue can increase metabolic rate, as you not only use up calories by being active, but your muscles use up lots of energy – even when you are not using them.

Having a high metabolic rate can help with achieving and maintaining a slim figure, however it will not make you immune to weight gain if your environment is not slim. Even people with 'fast metabolism' are not 'naturally' slim. If they overeat and don't do enough exercise they will put weight on just like everybody else. Many thin people may put their slim figures down to having a naturally fast metabolism, however it is extremely likely that they are also well-practised at being slim and burn up calories at a higher rate than others due to being more physically active than it first appears.

Metabolism –
how do we use up the calories?

Although being active uses more energy than resting, most of the calories that we burn (approximately 70%) are spent on just keeping us alive 24 hours a day, seven days a week. This is called our basal metabolic rate and is the minimum amount of energy that we would require if we didn't 'do' anything other than stay in bed and sleep all day and night. On top of that we use up energy in physical activity (approximately 20% of our total energy expenditure). We also burn calories digesting and processing our food and producing body heat. These functions account for the remaining 10% of total energy that we use up.

What have we learnt about slim people?

Although the vast majority of people assume that some people are naturally slimmer than others, this is not actually the case. There is always a lifestyle reason which can explain why somebody is a particular weight and very often this comes down to compensation.

Slim people stay slim, either by eating well and exercising lots, or by compensating for weight-gaining habits with other, weight-losing, habits. The real secrets are how they manage to do this without appearing to restrict their lifestyles considerably. Many people work hard at being slim, yet have very often managed to convince others (and maybe even themselves) that it is all easy. Compared to dieting, working at 'being slim' is not very hard at all, however, the reward for this effort is a slim figure.

So to recap what we have learnt in *Secret One*:

- your body weight is largely *not* genetic and can vary a lot depending on the environment that you create for yourself,

- you may have acquired your attitudes towards your weight at a young age, but these can change,

- even if you have always been overweight, you can learn how to be slim,

- your natural body shape does not prevent you from being slim,

- slim people have different attitudes and habits that ensure that they remain slim,

- most slim people have to put effort into being slim, and achieve a slim figure in return.

You may find that *Secret One* has really made you think carefully about how other people seem to have it all. Knowing that being slim doesn't just come naturally should make you feel a lot more positive about any weight issues that you may have. There are solutions, and they lie with the slim people who have become masters of their art. Just being aware that anyone can be slim – you can be slim – should give you the confidence to really go for it. Learn from the masters – use slim (and healthy) people as your inspiration!

The remaining *Thin Secrets* will help you to understand slim people better, and reassure you that it is a level playing field once you know the little tricks of the game. Learning the secrets of slim people may seem strange at first, but these people are experts at not gaining weight. The attitudes that slim people have ensure that they remain slim. Anyone can learn and apply the same approach, lose weight and maintain a slim figure. There is no natural advantage, but with the right way of thinking (and a small amount of effort), being slim is within anybody's reach. Spending a little time really getting to grips with the *Thin Secrets* will be worth it considering the reward of a slim figure for the rest of your life.

Secret Two

"Slim people have chosen to be slim"

This may sound like a very strange *Secret*. Surely everybody chooses to be slim, it's just that some people manage it and others don't?

For many people, their weight does not become an issue until there is too much of it. Many slim people do not watch their weight, or bother about what size their clothes are. So how are they choosing to be slim? Some are not. However, the ones that will remain slim for life – the ones that know the *Thin Secrets* – have chosen. They have already worked out the correlation between their lifestyle and their weight and whenever they notice a small weight change, or a difference in the way that their jeans fit them, they will take action to bring it all back under control. This is before there is even a hint of a weight issue. They have chosen not to ignore the small changes, as they know that many small changes eventually will add up. In order to stay slim, they have to choose to actively maintain their weight, rather than sit back and see what happens.

The rest of the slim people are the ones that are prone to weight gain, either now or in the future. Their current lifestyles are 'slim', but because they have not actively chosen to be slim, they risk putting weight on without really noticing when their lifestyle changes. They do not act on small changes – they may not even notice small changes. They are used to being slim, but because they have not made the decision to actively stay slim, they are very prone to future weight gain.

I was one of these people, until I made the decision that I was going to be slim. My childhood and teenage years had set me up nicely with some good, slim habits. My food decisions were not made by me and were mainly based around family meals or school dinners. I was also very active, with four to five hours of sport a week. I left home for university very much used to the idea that I was slim – it had just happened to me. I assumed that because I always had been slim, I didn't need to pay too much attention to my weight. I had not really made the link between my lifestyle and my weight, and it didn't even occur to me that I would have to watch my weight now that my lifestyle had changed. My eating habits changed and I did less exercise. Lo and behold, I put weight on – not a lot, and not enough to worry about, but still the penny didn't drop! With hind-sight, maybe I was relying on the possibility that somebody would tell me when I had put weight on, but as nobody did I rationalised that it wasn't really a problem.

After a while, I figured out that not only had I put weight on, but that I was still gaining weight. At the end of each term, I weighed a bit more than I did at the start of that term. My saving grace was going home for the vacations, where some of the damage done during term-time was reversed.

Although there was a general upward trend in my weight, I was not particularly worried about it. I was not very overweight. In fact, there was always someone else who was a lot bigger than me, which gave me false comfort. I justified it by telling myself that I was having fun at university, I would worry about dieting afterwards. I guess that deep down, I was hoping that it would somehow sort itself out.

About a year after I left university I bought my own set of weighing scales. I was shocked at the weight. I didn't feel any bigger than I had done the previous year, but the weight was still going on – I obviously was bigger. I had moved away from home permanently, so I no longer had those vacation opportunities, the months spent at home, to undo some of the damage.

At that point I had to admit to myself that the weight doesn't just go away if you ignore it. It was then that I decided that I was going to be a slim person. I had to make that choice. Dieting didn't seem to work for me and I couldn't rely on the fact that I had been slim previously to keep me slim in the future. I also couldn't hold on to the idea that I would somehow store up all the damage and go on one big diet when I needed to.

I started to watch what the people who stay thin did. I also took note of how my at-home habits and my new habits were different. I began to change my lifestyle gradually. As a result I lost weight. During that process I leant how to live like a slim person.

By choosing to be slim, I had made the decision to notice the small changes and to not let the excess weight creep-up on me again. If I had not chosen to be slim at that point, and just put it to the back of my mind, to deal with at another time, then I would probably be very overweight by now.

If I had chosen to be slim earlier, I would never have put the weight on in the first place, although I really learnt through experience that even slim people who overeat and do not do enough exercise will put weight on. As a consequence of making changes to my lifestyle, I have found a weight that I am happy with, which is relatively easy for me to maintain. It is still more work for me to stay slim than it is for me to gain weight, but I have chosen to be slim and so the small amount of effort is worth it. I know that in the short term, it would be an easier life to put weight on; however I would be saving myself up a problem for the future. Anybody can achieve the same thing and be slim by living a slim lifestyle.

In order to become a slim person, <u>you</u> must choose to be a slim person. This still may sound a bit funny. Yes, you may want to lose weight and have a slim figure, but it's not the same as choosing to live like a slim person. Deciding to be slim means accepting that you will have to make choices about your lifestyle, your eating habits and the amount of exercise that you do in order to achieve and maintain your new slim figure. Choosing to be slim also means believing that you can make it happen – which you can!

Staying slim requires a slim person's attitude

An important part of choosing to be slim means not putting the weight on in the first place. Okay, that might not be very much help if you already have weight that you wish to lose, but it is important to know as it is the mentality of someone who is slim for life.

Slim people, who have chosen to be slim, know that if they overeat and don't do sufficient exercise, they will gain weight. They choose to keep the balance right, most of the time, allowing themselves the odd indulgence, but at the same time, keeping an eye on things to check everything is still under control. So the doughnut at coffee-time, or the odd (rather large) meal out with an old friend, does not sabotage their weight control, as it is what they are doing most of the time that is important.

This does not fit in with most people's perception, which is that slim people do not need to bother with their weight and they can eat whatever they please. Fortunately, this is false and slim people are no different to anybody else. People who wish to remain slim need to choose to keep a close eye on their weight, or their figures. They avoid going down a route which will make them overweight, instead they choose to be slim. This does not mean that they miss out on life. Instead they enjoy a balanced lifestyle where the occasional indulgences are easily compensated for and will not add up to a disastrous effect on the waistline.

If a slim twenty-year-old begins to notice that they are putting weight on gradually, but takes no action, that is fine. In the short term, their weight will not be an issue. Let's say, for example, that this young person is gaining weight at the rate of two pounds per year. On most people, this is hardly noticeable at all. However, if they carry on at the same rate, then by the time that 'slim' person is 41, they will have gained three stones. By that point, they will certainly have noticed a weight gain, but will be so used to their lifestyle that they will probably continue to put weight on, unless they choose to do something about it. Now fast-forward to the time that 'slim' person is collecting their bus pass and the situation has deteriorated somewhat. Having put weight on at a steady, hardly noticeable, nothing-to-worry-about rate of just two pounds a year, that person, at age 65, will weigh a whopping six and a half stones more than they did at age twenty!

That's where deciding that you will not ignore a couple of pounds here or there becomes very important if you are to stay slim for life!

Notice the little changes and take immediate action

So how does knowing that slim people choose to be slim help *you* to lose weight? Saying, "don't put the weight on in the first place", may feel a little bit like closing the stable door after the horse has bolted – but trust me, it will still help you.

Firstly, it helps to know that once you reach your target weight, and you are a slim person, you need to choose to remain slim, otherwise it is likely that you will put the weight back on. Secondly, it helps to really get to grips with the accumulation factor. Knowing that a couple of pounds here and there can add up to stones eventually, helps to keep you motivated when losing weight, as well as giving you a good reason for not ignoring small weight gain. Every little bit of weight that you lose makes a contribution. Over time, all of those small contributions can add up to a lot of weight lost!

We have seen from *Secret One* that there is no such thing as a naturally slim person. Someone who has chosen to be slim has an advantage as they accept that they have to work at staying slim. The ones that are working hard without realising that it is perfectly normal can often feel like they are trying to swim against the current.

The fact that it is not widely known that being slim requires effort may be the fault of our society. A slim person cannot easily refuse a 'treat' saying, "I'm watching my weight," or, "I overdid it at the weekend, I should really cut back a bit this week". This can often draw negative attention from others who have either refused the treat because the diet does not 'allow' it, or had the treat and felt guilty. There may be an assumption that the slim person is attention seeking, or fishing for compliments, or even that the slim person is passing judgement on others. There is a general consensus that slim people can eat whatever they please – people do not realise that it is a life-choice to be slim.

It is not just the difference in weight which separates people, it is the decisions that they make. In general, dieters would love to have the treat, but can't because they are working hard on a diet. However, they are looking forward to the day when they are slim and can eat whatever they please. A slim person, on the other hand, knows that they cannot eat whatever they please without gaining weight. They have chosen to be slim, and therefore, every now and again, something has to give. In this example it was the treat. However, the following week they may well choose to have the treat, as they didn't overdo it that weekend, or it is the first treat they have had all week.

By choosing to be slim, you are taking the first steps toward making it happen. Having a very clear goal of a slim, gorgeous figure will help you to focus. It will then become easier to act to make it happen. You can be slim, if you decide that you want to be. A smoker who tries to quit because they feel like they ought to, will not be as successful as the smoker who quits because they actually want to. You may have dieted in the past because you felt that you should do. Instead decide to be slim, choose to be slim and want to be slim and you will have the best chance of success.

Although being slim requires you to make a choice, and it is some-times hard work, the better you are at it, the more enjoyable it can be. So, you can't eat whatever you want to, whenever you want to and do no exercise, but you can eat your favourite foods in moderation and still have a slim figure. You may even find that you enjoy eating your favourite foods more when they become occasional indulgences, because you can have these without feeling guilty.

You have to be aware of how your choices affect your weight and notice how the little things can quickly add up. Choosing to be slim is only the first part; once you have decided to be slim, you will have to make choices which reflect this. However, factoring 'being slim' into your decision-making can really help you to make more slim choices.

Knowing that you must choose to be slim is a huge step. It is very different from just wanting to be slim. Choosing to make something happen <u>for</u> you is a lot more powerful than just wanting it to happen <u>to</u> you.

Have you chosen to be slim?

You can open the door to a new approach to weight control simply by accepting that:

- nobody is naturally slim,

- being slim requires effort (but not as much as being on a diet),

- you need to choose to be slim,

- 'being slim' is not about denial and can be enjoyable, especially as the reward is a permanent slim figure.

Secret Three

"Being slim is a priority for slim people"

We have talked about how being slim does not come naturally to most people, and how you must consciously decide to be slim in order to avoid the weight creeping on without really noticing it. What does somebody do once they have 'chosen' to be a slim person? How do we go from decision to action?

Everybody has their own priorities in life. You may rank family, friends and having a job as priorities in life. For some people, having a nice house or car, or the latest gadget, is a priority and they are prepared to seek out a well paid job in order to have those things. If you decide that you wanted to find a partner, you would probably go out and meet people. Later on, you would put effort into your relationships in order to ensure that they were successful. Why should your weight be any different?

If you didn't make going to work a priority, you would soon find yourself out of a job. Likewise, if you ignored your boyfriend, you then couldn't expect to have a fulfilling relationship. You put effort into your relationship, your job and even your hobbies because they are important to you.

You may feel like being slim is important to you. At the same time though, you may not actually be investing much in being slim. Being slim, without putting in any effort, is like expecting a pay cheque at the end of the month when you didn't turn up for work. Going to work every day doesn't seem so bad when you think about getting paid. The easiest option of course is not to go to work – but obviously most people need the money.

It is the same with being slim. Some effort is required to remain slim, or to lose weight. Unfortunately, it doesn't just happen. However, if something is a priority for you – in that it will make you happier – then you don't mind putting a little bit of work in to achieve it.

If you have ever been on a diet to lose weight, then you will have temporarily made your weight a priority. At the start of the diet, you were likely to be making a lot of decisions based on the diet – and prioritising the rules of the diet ahead of other things, such as eating out. Maybe you prioritised eating certain types of food over others. Initially, the diet may have been very successful, resulting in weight loss. However, if it had not been a priority, then your weight would have remained the same. Imagine being on a diet, but not really caring about sticking to 'the rules' if other things came up. It would not work very well. You would not achieve the results that you wanted.

Slim people have made being slim a priority in their lives. They have chosen to not put weight on and they will prioritise aspects of their lifestyle that keep them slim. This may be certain eating habits, or exercise, and could include lots of little things, which will all add up.

I know someone who will rarely leave the house without a healthy snack with them. This means that they must prepare and pack the food (which they must previously have shopped for) before they go out. They do this because when they get hungry, they feel the need to find something to eat quite quickly. If they did not have something healthy with them, the chances are that they would pick up a chocolate bar, or a bag of crisps, maybe even a cheeseburger, to satisfy their hunger. That little bit of extra time that it takes to make a sandwich, or pack some fruit before leaving the house, is an example of making 'being slim' a priority. Initially, it requires some forward planning to make sure that the slim options are available, but once it becomes a habit to buy sandwich fillings or healthy snacks with the weekly shop the extra work becomes unnoticeable. It also often saves time finding a vending machine or a shop when out and may even save money too.

It doesn't sound like much, but if the snack was needed once or twice in a week, that is one or two fewer chocolate bars eaten. Little things add up, as the accumulation factor kicks in; that is 50-100 chocolate bars (or bags of crisps, or cheeseburgers) per year that have been replaced with healthier options! If lots of slim choices are made, they will very soon start to have a big effect.

It is important to note that if the snack is not needed then there is no requirement to eat it just because it is there.

To use a personal example of prioritising 'being slim', I have to plan my exercise into my day before I plan anything else. Obviously, I plan it at a time that I know won't interfere with my job. However, if I tried to fit it around my job, my social life, the weekly shop, taking my library books back, phoning my mother, balancing my chequebook etc., I would never do any exercise. I have to make exercise a priority over the other things, as I know I'll fit those things in anyway (if they are important). If I wait to see if I have any spare time left in my day, then I will never get round to doing any exercise at all. Being slim doesn't just happen, you have to make it happen.

If you want to be slim – make 'being slim' a priority

Living like a slim person, and being slim, will only happen for you if you make it a priority in your life. That's not to say that you need to give up the day job and just concentrate on being slim. Losing weight may be important to you, but other things in life can easily get in the way of that if you do not make 'being slim' a priority. Why put dealing with your weight on hold? The less damage that has already been done, the easier it is to fix. If you want to be slim, you must make it happen. One of the ways to achieve this is to make a healthy lifestyle – with a balanced diet and plenty of exercise – a priority for you. You will then become a healthy weight, and look slimmer.

Move 'being slim' up your list of priorities and see the difference that it makes. It will not get in the way of anything else in your life (anything important, that is). However it will give you a great sense that you are actively working towards losing weight. Make time every day to work on 'being slim' until it becomes a habit for you. It will keep you focused and you will soon see fantastic results. Later on in the book, we will see what habits you can adopt to help you to lose weight and become slim for life. By making it a priority to become slim, you will be able to easily change some of your habits that were keeping you trapped with weight issues. Move on to weight loss by making it a priority for you – today.

Secret Four

"Slim parents pass on 'slim' habits to their children"

Body weight, be it slim or overweight, appears to run in families. At first glance, this seems to strengthen the claim that your weight is genetic and that there is nothing you can do about it. However, we saw from the identical twin example earlier how much of an impact that 'environment' or lifestyle can have on weight, and this can affect whole families. This is fantastic news for anybody who is overweight, who has felt like they have been trapped. Your weight is not predetermined by your genetics – you can change your weight.

The reason that body weight appears to run in families is more to do with the lifestyles of all the family members being very similar, rather than genetics. Many of the habits and attitudes towards eating and exercise that you learnt when you were young have probably stayed with you, and had a huge impact on your adult weight. They are also likely to form the basis of what your children learn. If your parents didn't like doing a lot of exercise, the chances are that you have not learnt to enjoy exercise. You may very well pass a similar attitude onto your children. You may have learnt particular habits from a very young age and this may be the reason that you have gained weight. By accepting this you now have a wonderful opportunity to start to alter the way that you approach your weight, and change some of your lifelong habits. You can learn to think like a slim person and adopt a new slim environment for yourself. Break free from the old ways of thinking and pave the way for the new, 'slim' approach.

Karen

Karen had never been particularly slim. In fact she had been dieting almost constantly since she was a teenager, but always seemed to put any weight that she lost straight back on again. Now in her thirties, she was beginning to give up on the idea that she would ever be slim. Even though Karen did not like being overweight, she had always felt that it was quite natural for her, as none of the women in her family were slim. One day, Karen became so fed up with constantly dieting, but always being overweight that she started to wonder whether this was the way she wanted to spend her life; she was miserable. She rationalised that she must have inherited a tendency to gain weight, and that no amount of dieting would ever rid her of it. That evening, she ordered pizza – as of course she was going to get fat anyway, why delay the inevitable?

Okay, the story simplifies a very complex situation, but deliberately so to illustrate a point. Karen never really felt in control of her weight, and deep down, she always thought that one day she would get fat. She had inherited certain attitudes and habits from her family, such as a constant cycle of dieting and putting weight on again, which didn't help her to lose weight in the long run. Along with this she saw that her whole family were large and this made her believe that being overweight was inevitable for her. If we fast forward a few years then we would probably find that 'the inevitable' has caught up with Karen much quicker than she expected. It will seem to prove her theory, making her less likely to try and lose weight again. Although Karen did not choose to become fat, she did not choose to be slim either as she did not realise that she could. If she had known at eighteen that she was overweight because she had overweight habits, which she could change, the situation would have been very different. Learning to live like a slim person may not have given Karen the dramatic short-term results that she wanted from a diet, but there is no doubt that she would have benefited in the long term.

It is not too late for Karen to learn the "Thin Secrets", and it may prevent her children from going through the same thing.

Fortunately, being overweight is generally not genetic. There are some extremely rare genetic disorders, which can cause people to gain a lot of weight, but these are often diagnosed by a doctor at a young age. Therefore, being overweight for the vast majority of people is due to their lifestyles. Luckily this means that there is a lot that can be done to change our weight and that being overweight is not a life sentence. Being slim will not last for long if slim habits change significantly and it is the same for overweight habits.

Slim people may believe that they have inherited 'good genes' from their parents; however it is much more likely that they have inherited good habits. They are also much more likely to have slim children, if they pass on those slim habits and attitudes. If you have children at home, then by learning to have a slim way of thinking, you could change not only your future weight, but you will also be well on the way to ensuring that your kids will learn to be slim too.

These slim parents have worked out how to stay slim and it is a real advantage for the children to learn it from a young age. However, just because everybody at home was slim, it doesn't mean that it will always be that way. Many young adults leave home and gain weight. Some can also lose weight, but this doesn't happen nearly so often! This is because there have been significant changes to their lifestyles and the habits that kept them slim at home have changed. Maybe they only have to look after themselves and find it easier to buy convenience foods than to cook for one. Other habits may also change, like drinking more alcohol and going out for dinner more often which will inevitably lead to weight gain.

However, it is not only the kids who leave home that have to worry about gaining weight. The effect of an empty nest may cause significant lifestyle changes to the parents. Suddenly going from feeding a whole family and shopping for several, to just shopping and cooking for one or two can take a bit of adjustment. A change like this is bound to affect habits and lifestyle and consequently weight.

Even if you were not brought up in a 'slim' family environment, and it is likely that you have several learnt habits that have been responsible for you gaining weight, it is still possible to learn how to be slim. You can be a slim person, even if you have never been slim before. You can adopt a 'slim' approach towards your weight and begin to change your environment. Your lifestyle habits will change and have a huge impact on your weight. Not only will you lose weight but you will also ensure that you don't put any back on again. In doing so you may well inspire the rest of the family to adopt the new 'slim' approach!

Break free from attitudes that hold you back from weight loss!

Secret Five

"Your weight will always reflect your overall lifestyle"

Have you ever found that your weight can remain fairly constant for quite a long period of time?

Many people hit a plateau of a particular weight that stays roughly the same for a long time. If this is the case you can get quite used to your weight. You can go on holiday and your weight does not really change, you could be ill for a few days and your weight doesn't really change. You could even diet for a few weeks, but as soon as you stop, your weight goes back up to what it was before. We then start to think that this is the weight that we are always going to be. It hasn't changed; therefore it must be a natural weight for our body type, right? Wrong! In actual fact, this is just our 'lifestyle weight'.

Your weight may seem to be constant, but it is not. It is linked to your lifestyle. The reason that your weight can stay the same for a long time is because your lifestyle can stay the same for a long time. So a few days off from your normal routine may cause a small alteration in your weight, but as soon as you go back to 'normal' your weight will go back to 'normal'. Have you ever found that you have lost weight, maybe through dieting, and then very quickly gone back to the weight that you were previously?

Slim people stay slim because they lead a slim lifestyle; this is their normal. They have the balance right between the amount of energy they consume and the amount that they use up so they do not put weight on. They have a slim lifestyle MOST of the time. Your weight will always reflect your lifestyle and therefore the best way to achieve a slim and healthy weight is to have a healthy lifestyle, MOST of the time.

This can help to explain why we can put weight on, or lose weight, when something changes in our lives. Changes can include getting a new job, moving house, starting or ending a relationship, or going through a period of stress, or bereavement. These life events are bound to have an impact on our lifestyle – what we eat, when we eat, how much we eat and how much exercise we do. This is why our weight changes. Small changes to your lifestyle bring about small changes in your weight. If you make a lot of small changes, over time this can add up to a significant change in weight. If your diet stayed the same and you started to do a bit more exercise, then you would gradually lose some weight.

There will be a little bit of delay between making changes to your lifestyle and seeing results. A few days of making changes and then reverting back to normal will have very little impact and will just leave you frustrated. Your weight will very quickly go back to normal again. However, if you make permanent changes to your lifestyle, the weight loss that occurs as a result will also be permanent. You will continue to lose weight until you reach your new lifestyle weight. That is until there is a new balance, between the amount of energy that you take in and the amount that you use up.

You will maintain that weight for as long as you maintain that lifestyle. So if your lifestyle became reasonably healthy – a balanced diet, with exercise – your weight will change to reflect this new lifestyle and you will have a healthy weight and look slimmer.

If you change your lifestyle, your weight will change

Once you have chosen to be slim, and made 'being slim' a priority, you can begin to start choosing and prioritising aspects of your lifestyle which will help you achieve this. Your weight will change to reflect the changes in your lifestyle.

What is a healthy weight to aim for?

As we saw earlier, being slim and being healthy are not necessarily the same thing. I personally would rather be a little bit overweight and healthy, than slim and unhealthy. Fortunately, you can have it both ways; you can be slim AND healthy. If you aim for a healthy lifestyle, a healthy weight will follow. A good indication of whether you have a healthy weight comes from calculating your Body Mass Index (BMI). At the back of this book you will find a table with your ideal weight range and a formula to calculate your own BMI (alternatively you can use the BMI calculator on our website www.thinsecrets.com). If you have a BMI between 20 and 25, then you are within a healthy weight range for your height. Anything above this and you need to consider losing a bit of weight. If your BMI is below 20, you should not be trying to lose weight.

It is important to be healthy
as well as slim!

The healthy BMI of 20–25 corresponds to a wide range of weights so all body types are accounted for (except *very* athletic types and possibly exceptionally tall people). Therefore, one person with a BMI of 22 may look slimmer than someone else with the same BMI, depending on their body types. However, both people will be healthy weights for their heights.

It is fine to have a healthy BMI and want to lose weight, just as long as you do not try to achieve a weight that would lower your BMI to an unhealthy figure. For very thin people, the health risks can be just as serious as being overweight.

Have realistic expectations

There are very few supermodels in the world – these are very tall women who are very thin. So if you are only 5'1" you may never look like a supermodel, however you can still be slim and gorgeous like many pint-sized pop stars! However the slimness that I describe in this book is within anybody's reach, and is the normal, everyday type of slim. Anyone aiming to be a size 6 is going a little bit too far in my opinion. We are not talking about people who are slim enough to make a living out of wearing clothes. Supermodels get paid a fortune because they have something a bit different – they were 'spotted' as tall, slim teenagers, with pretty faces, and given jobs that required them to stay very thin. That pressure to stay thin has probably ensured that they did.

These women have to put a huge amount of effort into staying very thin. I'm sure they are working on it all day, every day, mainly by being extremely careful about what they eat. If a supermodel ate too much of the 'wrong' sorts of food and did no exercise, they would put weight on, like any other slim person. They would probably also lose their jobs! They are the ultimate examples of women who know what it is that keeps them slim, and they work very hard to maintain it.

There is no point in aiming to be that thin, and nobody is expecting you to. The slimmer you want to be, the more of an impact it will have on your lifestyle. How much of a balance do you want to achieve between your lifestyle and your weight? Bear in mind that healthily slim is achievable with a 'normal' and enjoyable lifestyle, *very thin* requires some major sacrifices!

The slimmer you wish to be, the harder that you will have to work to get there. Once you get there, if you stop working at it you will put weight on again, as your weight will always reflect your lifestyle. The good news is that a healthy weight is much easier to maintain than being underweight, and it often looks much better. Aiming for a healthy weight means that you can maintain a healthy relationship with food and still treat yourself occasionally. In addition you will still look slim. Why not aim for a healthy weight and a nice balance in your life-style? This means that you can be healthily slim, and still eat cake (occasionally)!

Being slim requires a whole lifestyle approach

So we now know that our normal weight is in fact our lifestyle weight and that our weight changes when our lifestyle changes. Slim people keep their weight fairly constant by having a fairly constant balance between the amount of energy that they are consuming and the amount that they are using up. This will be different for everyone; some people may eat a lot of food, but also do a lot of exercise. Others will not eat very much at all, and be fairly sedentary.

How does metabolism fit in?

If your daily energy needs (metabolic rate) and the amount of energy that you take in through food and drink are in balance then your weight will remain constant.[1] If your lifestyle changes then your energy intake will probably change, but your metabolic rate can also change.

If someone was consuming more calories than they needed, they would begin to put on weight. This is because the extra energy is being stored as fat. As the body gets heavier more energy is required to do everyday activities such as walking and climbing stairs (metabolic rate increases). Eventually the energy required by the bigger body will equal the energy that person is regularly consuming, and there will be no excess energy left to be stored. When this happens, that person will

1   If you want to calculate your approximate metabolic rate then go to our website www.thinsecrets.com

not put any more weight on as they are not using up any more or any less energy than they are taking in.

There are other factors which can affect metabolic rate:

How age affects metabolic rate ...

A lightly active 25 year old who is 5'4" tall, and weighs 9 stones would require approximately 1911 calories per day to maintain her weight. This is her metabolic rate. At age 45 (assuming that she was equally active and still weighed 9 stones) she would require only 1782 calories to maintain the same weight. Therefore, the same woman needs 129 fewer calories per day at 45 than she did at 25 due to her metabolic rate change. This is approximately the number of calories in half a standard chocolate bar.

How weight affects metabolic rate ...

Let's go back to that 25 year old who requires 1911 calories per day. If she were to gain two stones in weight (while still being lightly active), then her metabolic rate would have increased to 2073 calories per day. That is how many calories would be needed everyday to maintain her new weight. If she regularly ate fewer calories, she would lose weight. Taken the other way, if this 9 stone woman regularly ate 2073 calories, she would slowly gain weight until she reached approximately 11 stone! Again, this is only just over half a chocolate bar extra a day.

How physical activity affects metabolic rate ...

If the same woman (weighing 9 stones at age 25) were to become more active and, instead of lightly exercising once a week, starts moderately exercising three times a week, her metabolic rate would increase from 1911 to 2154 calories per day. However, if her diet remained the same and she was still only taking in 1911 calories per day she would lose weight as she is using up more energy than she is providing her body with.

Problems arise when someone regularly consumes a huge amount of *excess* energy. They would gain a lot of weight before their body's energy needs increased enough to match what was being provided. Weight will stabilise eventually, but not until that person is very heavy. Somebody who is regularly eating a large amount can get used to having that much food (even though it is more than the body actually requires). They may then feel that they need to have even more food to feel satisfied and it can be very difficult to cut down.

When a person's weight is constant, a change such as eating fewer calories or using up more energy though exercise will cause weight loss. This is because the body has to use some of its energy reserves to make up for the shortfall and this comes from fat stores around the body.

If you have ever hit a plateau in your weight, it is because your energy consumption (calories eaten) and your energy requirements (metabolic rate) have been in balance. If this weight is higher than you would like then you need to tip the balance in your favour. The way to lose weight is to either reduce you energy intake, or to increase the amount you use through exercise (or a combination of both). This does not mean that you have to starve yourself, or spend hours in the gym. It can be achieved very easily with lots of small changes to your lifestyle, which over time will have a huge impact on your weight.

If someone has been gaining weight for a number of weeks or months, then it is safe to assume that their weight has not yet caught up with their lifestyle. Their energy in and energy out are not yet in balance; there is always more energy than needed and this is constantly being stored as fat. This person may find that reducing their calorie intake may only slow the rate at which they gain weight for a little while as the energy balance was not right to begin with. It may take a bit longer until they see a drop in weight as the changes in their lifestyle have only acted to bring the energy more into balance in the first instance.

Why do some people lose weight quickly?

Have you ever been to a slimming club and found that other people have lost weight more quickly than you, even though you have been trying very hard? This may be because you did not have a constant weight when you started the diet. If you had been steadily gaining weight, you may not yet have reached the energy balance. The initial period of the diet may have been spent achieving a balance to start maintaining a weight. In the meantime you may have felt quite fed up with seeming to make little progress. In reality you may have avoided gaining more weight (which is a good thing). Unfortunately, with dieting there are no rewards for weight maintenance.

This helps to explain why some people can lose weight more quickly than others.

If you have a steady lifestyle weight, then you are in a very good position to start making lifestyle changes that will bring about a gradual reduction in your weight. If you are still gaining weight, then you can also make changes that will bring your weight down, however it may be a while before you see the effect as pounds lost on the scales. It will happen though, just stick with it.

Although a great deal of emphasis has been put on calorie intake and calorie requirements here, it does not follow that the only way to lose weight is to strictly count calories. The examples given were to illustrate how different lifestyle factors, such as exercise, can have a real effect on weight. It is not necessary to know your metabolic rate, or memorise the number of calories each food contains. However it helps to be aware of why it becomes more difficult to maintain body weight as we age, or why two people can follow exactly the same diet and one loses weight quicker than the other.

Being slim requires a slim lifestyle
MOST of the time

It is important to remember that muscle weighs more than fat, so weight should not be your only measure. You can be extremely fit, healthy and slim, but still weigh more than someone who looks larger if you have more muscle mass than they do. So if you started to tip the energy balance, however simultaneously started to tone up your muscles, it is possible that you would gain weight temporarily, because of the extra muscle. Your weight may increase even though you are losing fat and slimming down! Don't worry about this though as muscle tissue uses up a lot of energy – which is why having more muscle increases your metabolic rate. Fat uses up little energy, although it does require extra energy to lug it around all day!

The whole lifestyle approach to being slim does not mean that you have to drastically change your whole lifestyle. What it does mean is that your weight will reflect your whole lifestyle so if you spend two weeks on a diet it is unlikely that you will see any significant long-term changes. However, if you aim to have a slim lifestyle, MOST of the time, this should have a huge impact on your weight, ensuring that you become slim.

If you feel like you need to lose weight, then making changes to your lifestyle will help to bring this about. There is no point trying for a week or two to become slim permanently. However, if you incorporate small changes into your lifestyle, gradually and slowly, you will find that your body weight will alter as your weight comes into balance. We will be looking at how you can begin to introduce 'slim' habits into your routine later on in the book.

Instead of concentrating on just losing weight, focus instead on getting your energy balance to work in your favour. Small lifestyle changes can add up to a big difference in the energy equilibrium, which will in turn lead to a change in weight. If your current lifestyle caused you to gain the weight, why not adopt a different lifestyle to reverse the trend? Being slim takes some effort, but adapting your lifestyle to ensure you remain slim is much easier than trying to lose weight by dieting.

When exercise and healthy living are a high priority, weight will not be an issue

Secret Six

"Dieting does not work in the long term"

We have all heard the old adage "dieting makes you fat". That statement may be a little bit of an exaggeration; however dieting is not the solution to staying slim permanently. As dieting can be a pretty rotten process, it should be music to the ears to know that there are other, more successful ways to ensure weight loss.

You can lose weight without dieting

Your weight will always reflect your lifestyle. What dieting does is provide a temporary lifestyle which has been designed to result in weight loss, and for a while, weight management becomes a priority in your life. Diets usually focus on a low calorie intake, caused by eating only certain types of food, or eating a lot less than you are used to. This temporary lifestyle is not sustainable in the long term, due to the fact that it is extremely hard work and generally fairly miserable. In addition, there is absolutely no incentive to stay on the diet once you have reached your target weight.

Dieting may result in fantastic weight loss and in that respect can be extremely effective. However, dieting does not deal with our normal lifestyle. It is this 'normal' lifestyle which determines our 'normal' weight, so once the diet has finished, our weight will start to creep back up until we are back to the same weight we were before the diet. This again will make us feel like we are 'naturally' an overweight person, that our 'natural' weight is something set in stone that we cannot have very much influence over. Why put yourself through all this?

Some diets are more in tune with a healthy lifestyle than others. Generally the ones that recommend eating less fat and cutting down on sugar are better options than the ones which encourage a very restrictive calorie intake, or the removal of whole food groups from all of your meals. The latter option requires quite dramatic changes to your lifestyle and this is probably why people report quite dramatic initial results. In the long term though, those results are not sustainable as the lifestyle (restrictive diet) that produced them is not sustainable. So if the best diets are based around a healthy lifestyle, how come we need to go on a diet to lose weight – why not just aim for a healthier lifestyle?

To start with, many people are used to the idea that if you want to lose weight, you should go on a diet. Just trying to be healthier doesn't seem to be the first option for a lot of people for some reason. Maybe it is to do with not having the confidence to go it alone? Maybe it's to escape peer pressure with, "I'm on a diet," being the only excuse that you can get away with for refusing to eat 'bad' foods? Some people don't particularly like preparing or eating healthy foods, so they will always get that feeling of hardship that comes with being on diet. Well, here's the good news. By adopting a 'slim' approach to weight loss, you will be able to choose what you do. You will not have to obey the rules of the diet, you can set your own pace.

Personally, I think the need to diet is down to control. When you go on a diet, you hand over control of what you eat to that diet plan. True, it's up to you to buy, cook and eat what you are supposed to, but you are just going through the motions. On a diet, you do not have to make decisions about what to eat and when – you just follow instructions. That means that although you do as the diet requires, you can hate the diet at the same time.

You are effectively putting your life on hold while you are on a diet. It can begin to feel like you have two alternate states of existence – being 'on' the diet and being 'off' the diet. When you are on the diet, you have to eat what you should. You are not allowed to eat 'bad' foods. When you aren't on the diet, you can eat 'bad' food. This split personality approach to weight loss will not give you the best results, as you are constantly fighting with yourself.

Dieting removes our feeling of control

Dieting teaches us to have quite deep negative associations with certain foods, and we will feel guilty about eating them. There are foods that can cause weight gain but there are no 'bad foods'. As the diet is based on self-denial, you may begin to obsess about the very foods that you are not 'allowed'. You may start to resent the diet, and eventually rebel against the diet.

So it doesn't matter how close the diet is to a healthy lifestyle, because if you feel restricted by the diet, you want to rebel against it. You want to eat 'bad' foods, just because you are not allowed to do so on the diet. Once you have 'suffered' through weeks of dieting, the prospect of living a healthy lifestyle permanently feels like it would be a prison sentence. That is the dieting mentality. Foods are often categorised as 'good' or 'bad', 'allowed' or 'forbidden'.

With a lifestyle approach, no food is banned. That means that you can eat anything that you want to, in moderation, as part of a balanced diet. The key word is balance. If there is equilibrium between the amount of energy that you take in (as calories) and the amount that you use up, your weight will remain constant, as there is no excess energy to be converted into fat for storage. There is also no requirement to use up any of your stored fat. If you tip the balance one way and begin to use up more energy than you have taken in, your body will begin to use up its supply of stored fat to provide for the shortfall.

The chances are that while you have been living your current life-style, you have been consuming more energy than your body needs and that extra energy has been stored as fat. So the most effective way of losing weight is to tip the energy balance in your favour. This is the principle that most diets work on. However, dieting often only takes into account what you eat, thereby ignoring 50 % of the balance.

Diets only provide a temporary solution to an ongoing problem

The most effective way of losing weight is to reduce the amount of excess energy that you consume and increase the amount that you use up through physical activity at the same time. This will alter the life-style/weight balance more quickly and effectively. The greater the difference between 'energy in' and 'energy out', then the more impressive the weight change will be. Dieting alone does not look at the bigger picture and it does not take into account that you do not want to feel restricted when it comes to what you can eat.

Although it may require some effort from you initially to change your lifestyle habits, it is the best thing that you can do. A whole lifestyle approach to weight loss is far more successful than dieting in the long term.

The expectation to diet leads to weight gain

Women are likely to diet at certain times of the year, particularly before they go on holiday, whereas men are more likely to attempt to lose weight when they feel that they need to.[2] In the approach to the summer holidays, women's magazines are full of advice to help us to achieve our "bikini body in just 2 weeks," or something similar. New

2   Taken from a survey of randomly selected students asked to list which times of the year that they were more likely to attempt to lose weight.

Year is also a traditional diet time. How many people do you know who make a New Year's resolution to lose weight, EVERY SINGLE YEAR? Year after year people go on diets to lose weight – some fail, some succeed, but lots of them will be dieting again at the same time next year! Does this ever happen to you?

Slim people do not diet at certain times of the year. They regulate their weight, by leading a slim lifestyle, and are rewarded with a slim body all year round. This is the lifestyle that they are used to, so although it may seem easier to just ignore the desire to be slim and begin to put weight on, the biannual diet that has to compensate for it is hard work and miserable, and is not guaranteed to make up for all the weight gained in between times.

If you are in the habit of dieting at certain times of year then you may actually be setting yourself up to NEED to diet again. Spending two weeks trying to slim down for your summer holiday makes it MORE likely that you will overindulge, and rebel against the restrictiveness of the diet whilst you are on holiday. If you are lucky, you will come back from holiday exactly the same weight as you were a month before you left. If you are unlucky, you will have gained a bit of weight. You will then go back to your normal lifestyle, which will mean that you will regain your normal weight, thereby setting yourself up for the same cycle of dieting/overindulging next year.

Dieting can become a bad habit

Living like a slim person, you will not feel the need to slim down before a holiday, and therefore won't feel the need to cram your whole year's worth of overindulgence into a two week break. If you do overindulge a little bit on holiday then you may put on a little bit of weight, but you will be aware of how you can compensate afterwards. Your weight will always reflect your lifestyle, and as long as you make an effort to have a slim lifestyle you will quite soon have undone any damage.

The same thing can happen at New Year, but in reverse. The expectation of always dieting during January (in combination with the credit card bills and the short cold days), can make you overcompensate at Christmas. 'Knowing' that you will diet can tempt you into overdoing it. After all what does it matter if you put on a few extra pounds – you'll be dieting anyway, right?

Have you ever said to yourself on a Saturday night, "the diet starts on Monday", and then had a second helping of food which would be forbidden on the diet? The expectation to diet can actually result in us putting extra weight on, as we try to 'stock-up' before the diet starts.

This is another reason why dieting does not work in the long term. Instead of focusing on what we are trying to achieve – which is to be slim – we get bogged down with the restrictiveness of the diet. We rebel against the diet, or the expectation of the upcoming diet, and we sabotage our ultimate goal. We may feel like we have won a victory over the diet, but we are biting our noses off to spite our faces. At the end of the day, if the idea of going on a diet makes you want to reach for the chocolate, then do not go on a diet. If you want to be slim, choose to be slim, prioritise the things that will help you achieve it, and enjoy it along the way, by keeping some of the habits which you enjoy (such as the occasional chocolate bar). The results may take a little longer than they might on a fad diet, but in the meantime you will be enjoying life, and be far less likely to revert back to weight-gaining habits.

Instead of looking at dieting for a solution to our weight problem, we should be looking at our lifestyles. If our normal weight is more than we would like it to be, then we can assume that our normal lifestyle is making us fat. We need to slim down our lifestyles, in order to slim down our weight. Ignoring our normal lifestyle for a while, and replacing it with a diet, is only a temporary fix – and not a very pleasant one at that. If we get into slim habits, which persist long after the excess weight has disappeared, then we will be well on the way to being slim

– permanently. We need to let go of the attitude that the only way to be slim is to diet. Slim people have habits that keep them slim; they do not need to diet. If you can develop and maintain a slim lifestyle then you will never again have to diet.

Take a moment to pause and imagine yourself going on holiday without having been on a diet beforehand. Instead of feeling self-conscious on the beach you will be confidently showing off your slim figure in a new bikini. Making a few permanent changes to the way you approach your weight, and incorporating slim habits into your lifestyle will mean that you never again have to diet for any occasion. Not only that, but maintaining your weight requires much less effort overall than yo-yo dieting. If you think and act like a slim person permanently, you will always have a slim figure to show for it. Being slim is worth never going on a diet again for!

Secret Seven

"There is no holiday from 'being slim'!"

Hopefully your new slim attitude is beginning to take hold and you are raring to go ahead and start to live a slim and healthy lifestyle. If you adopt a whole lifestyle approach, you will find that making slim choices fits into your normal routine. It won't always be effortless, but it gets easier the more you are in the habit of doing so. But what happens when you go on holiday and take a break from your normal routine? What happens if you just have a few days off from a slim lifestyle? Can you take a holiday from 'being slim'? The answer is yes ... and no.

Slim people often have a break from making slim choices – the secret to staying slim comes in the 'compensation' that occurs around this. For example, having a normal sized, but healthy breakfast and lunch before an indulgent dinner, and then having three very healthy meals the following day, should more than compensate for the big dinner, in someone who is MAINTAINING their weight. For someone who wanted to lose weight, the compensation period would probably need to be more substantial than this.

Likewise, if the 'indulgence' was spread over a whole weekend, then a slim person may compensate all week to get back to their starting point again. By compensating, I do not mean dieting, but making that extra effort to be healthy and not to overeat. Just enough to bring everything back into balance again. That balance results in staying slim – it is worth it to not get carried away and begin to put on weight.

Another strategy would be not to compensate with eating, but to do more exercise. In fact, people who do a lot of exercise may find that they eat even more food to provide them with the energy that they require. The best fuels for exercise are high in carbohydrates and low in fat and sugar (increased exercise is not a good excuse for eating badly!). Obviously the fastest way to lose weight would be to eat healthily and exercise.

So in answer to the above question – yes, you can have time off from living like a slim person, but that time off will need to be compensated for in some way to avoid putting weight on. So by all means really enjoy your Christmas dinner, but go easy on Christmas Eve and Boxing day to compensate. Treat yourself on your birthday, but go easy for a few days afterwards. A short break from slim habits, if compensated for in some way, will not have too much of an effect on overall weight. This is why you will be able to enjoy the occasional treats, guilt-free and still not put weight on overall.

Learn to indulge guilt-free

What we have discussed so far relates to short periods of time off from 'being slim'. Indulging in moderation is fine; you may gain a pound or two as a result, but you can compensate for it easily. However, can you take a two week holiday from being slim? Not without putting some weight on. Remember that it is much easier to gain weight than to lose it. Being slim is a lifestyle choice – if you choose not to live like a slim person, you will put weight on. By all means have a two week holiday and indulge every single day, just be prepared for the fact that (like everybody else) if you overeat, or eat unhealthily, and fail to do sufficient exercise, you will gain weight.

The advantage of all this is that if you don't ever take much of a holiday from being slim, you will never take a break from looking slim either. You can have a fabulous figure all year round by living like a slim person.

Being slim is a way of life

Secret Eight
"Slim people are in control of their weight"

Have you ever wanted to feel more in control of your weight? You can be. Slim people are in control of their weight and that is NOT BECAUSE they are slim – it is WHY they are slim. Dieters often feel like they are not in control of their weight, especially after a week of intense dieting and no weight loss. Others can feel like their weight is just something that happens to them, they try to control it but don't quite manage to. Slim people focus less on controlling weight and more on controlling the factors which influence weight – you've guessed it – lifestyle! By mastering a 'slim' lifestyle, in turn, they have control over their weight.

Slim people are slim because they have worked out how to have that control; they have chosen to stay slim and therefore prioritise what they need to do in order to stay slim. Being in control gives you more confidence to know that you can change your weight. It is easy to decide that you are going to lose weight, but you don't just wake up one morning having lost seven pounds. What you can do instead is to make small changes to what you eat and drink, and how much you exercise, and as a result of that you will lose weight. This is because your weight will always reflect your lifestyle. After a while, your body will have adjusted to the small changes, and you may find that you have lost the desired seven pounds. If you have not, you may need to make some more changes to lose a little more weight; until you reach a weight – and a lifestyle – that you are comfortable with. Then it is time to look again at your lifestyle – because if you go back to the way you were before, you will very quickly put those pounds back on.

If you wish to be seven pounds less than you are now, you not only have to make an effort to get there, you will have to actively maintain it, with a lifestyle that has altered sufficiently, to avoid putting the weight back on. Slim people control their weight by making minor adjustments to their lifestyles when they wish to make small changes to their weight.

Adopting 'slim' attitudes will let you feel in control of your weight

The confidence to relax and feel in control of your weight will come when the attitudes that we have discussed previously have really taken hold. In addition, when you begin to see favourable results from just a few small lifestyle changes, you will know that you are really on the road to being in complete control of your weight.

Secret Nine

"The key lies in choice, but first you must accept your weight"

When it comes to being slim, there is very little luck involved. Okay, some people are lucky in that they realise earlier on in life what they need to do in order to be slim. This may be because they learnt from their parents, or at a young age, and this has kept them slim. Those people definitely have an advantage as they know that they CAN control their weight. This acceptance that we really do have the power to control our weight may not come easily. Once you have it though there will be no stopping you!

Previously, you may have thought that you had chosen to be slim, but it didn't really work out for you. This may be because we have spent years telling ourselves that we are not naturally slim, or that we are just big-boned, or maybe even denying to ourselves that our weight was ever an issue. Does any of this sound familiar? This kind of thinking may prevent you from losing weight (like it used to for me). However once you have accepted your weight, and accepted that you can control your weight, there are no obstacles left.

As well as not really believing that we can ever be slim, previous attempts at weight loss may have been less successful than we would have liked (or we have lost weight only to put it all back on again). No wonder that the confidence we need to start to change our habits and lifestyle may need a bit of a pick-me-up.

The good news is that you can work on accepting your weight. You can learn how to think like a slim person, and make decisions that reinforce the fact that being slim is a priority for you. It is the choices that you make that will help you lose weight and keep you slim. It is not genetics, or luck, or being on the 'right' diet. We will be working on accepting our weight more in the next section of the book.

To become slim you must live like a slim person. As well as choosing to be slim, you must make choices about your lifestyle. This includes all the small daily decisions about what to eat, and whether to exercise. Some of these choices will be easy, some will be more difficult. All of them will add up though, little by little. Eventually you will be so used to making lots of slim choices they seem to come naturally to you, but only of course if being slim is a priority for you. Your weight will change to catch up with your lifestyle. You WILL be a slim person, if you lead a slim lifestyle.

You CAN be that person who chooses to eat a huge dinner every once in a while, and smile to yourself, as the people around you wonder how it is that you stay so slim, with seemingly no effort whatsoever. You CAN be the one who can have the cake at coffee-time guilt-free while your colleagues moan about their restrictive diets. You can also choose whether you keep your secrets to yourself or whether you tell them that the reason you can eat cake guilt-free is that you live like a slim person MOST of the time. It is the choices that you make most of the time that will keep you slim.

It is up to you to choose. You can choose to accept your weight, choose to be slim, choose to make it a priority, and achieve it by a whole lifestyle approach. It can be tough to accept that you may need to change in order to successfully lose weight. This is both the easiest and the hardest part of truly becoming a slim person. Whilst it does not require any physical effort (the easy part), it may require a change in attitudes that can be very deep rooted.

The rest of this book is devoted to helping you to achieve it.

What now?
How do I use the Thin Secrets?

The *Thin Secrets* will help you to lose weight. *Thin Secrets* give you the confidence to know that, if you choose to, you can be slim, regardless of whether you have ever been slim in the past. It will require some effort and a bit of hard work on your part, but no more than it does for anybody else.

Slim people make tough choices, they prioritise being slim over some, but not all, of the pleasures that can come from eating indulgently. However, they also get the satisfaction of knowing that they are in control of their weight. They can relax as they do not need to slim down for any occasion, they will be slim permanently. Very well-practised slim people do not feel restricted by a slim lifestyle, it is their normal. However it does ensure that, when they do indulge, they can do so without any guilt.

The next section of the book shifts the focus away from slim people for a while. We will explore some very common ways of thinking which can be a barrier to weight loss. Being able to identify these will help you to accept your weight, and accept that you can change your weight. Later on, we can see how the old way of thinking can hinder our new 'slim' thinking, before we go on looking at a whole lifestyle approach to weight loss and staying slim.

Just accept it
Who is in control?

If you are overweight, it can sometimes feel like your excess weight has a lot of control over you. 'The weight' may be stopping you from wearing clothes that you want to wear, 'the weight' may be preventing you from being confident about yourself, 'the weight' has probably affected your mood at some point or another. It is very easy to let 'the weight' become the enemy, which gives it an awful lot of power. Maybe you are putting some things on hold until 'the weight' goes away. Does any of this sound familiar? Well, the good news is that you can make 'the weight' go away (the excess weight that is!), but first of all you have to regain the control that it has had over you and start thinking like a slim person.

Let's face it, we don't like 'the weight', and most of us just wish we could wave a magic wand and make it go away. However, instead of declaring loudly "I don't like being overweight, I am going to do everything in my power to change", what we often do is justify the weight, or become defensive about it. This is a perfectly natural reaction and many people do it. At times, even when we are thoroughly fed up about being overweight, we will go into self-destruct mode by simultaneously overeating AND making excuses about it AND feeling guilty. This can have a huge negative impact on our self-esteem and it prevents us from *accepting* our weight. Accepting our situation lets us go on to choosing and prioritising 'being slim'.

Accepting your weight can be tough. It may require you to let go of old attitudes and really extend your comfort zone. In the end though, it may make you a little bit happier about your weight – whatever it may be.

We do not need to justify our weight

When we try to justify our weight to ourselves, or to other people, we are actually providing 'the weight' with a seemingly valid reason for being there. Over time, we have developed some very nice justifications and defensive behaviours which we use when we feel like we are being judged or criticised. Not only that, but our friends and our family have been helping us to justify our weight, motivated by the good intention of making us feel better about ourselves. This is admirable; however in the long run, it does not give us any reason to change and 'the weight' stays.

First of all, you do not have to justify or defend your weight to anybody! Secondly, it is very important to realise that statements which justify or defend excess weight are actually keeping you trapped by a feeling of helplessness. In order to move on to successful, permanent weight loss you must recognise that these statements were giving 'the weight' too much control over you. We cannot accept our weight, and accept that we can change our weight, when we are trying very hard to justify it!

I have written a few of the more common 'False justification statements' in the next panel. There are probably plenty more that you have heard. Have a think and maybe add some more of your own.

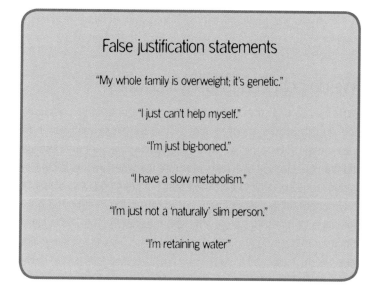

False justification statements

"My whole family is overweight; it's genetic."

"I just can't help myself."

"I'm just big-boned."

"I have a slow metabolism."

"I'm just not a 'naturally' slim person."

"I'm retaining water"

Very few people are confident enough to never feel like they have to justify themselves at some point or another. Not only do we justify our weight when we feel we are being judged but we can even do it when we are being complimented. In the past, if people asked me if I had lost weight, I used to reply that it was probably down to stress, or the new job. I know now that deep down, I was avoiding accepting the responsibility that I had over my weight, and playing-along with the popular belief that weight loss/gain was something that just happened to you, without you really having very much control over it. I was trying to distance myself from accepting the active role that I had in personal weight control.

The tendency to justify our weight has probably been learnt, maybe from our parents, maybe from our friends. It appears to be quite a usual thing to do in our society. As a consequence, many people have never been taught, or never really believed that they could have very much control over their weight. Instead, without them really knowing about it, the sense of control has been 'taken away' from them. How can you accept control over your weight when there are so many external factors working against you? These false justifications need to be removed.

If we regularly use these kinds of reasons to justify our weight then we are really holding ourselves back from weight loss. This is because we have convinced ourselves deep down that we will never be slim because something – that we cannot change – is keeping us the way we are. All of these statements are trying to lay the blame for excess weight with forces which are beyond our control. The need to blame is understandable; however, it can be quite destructive. Blame doesn't solve anything. Although justifications may temporarily help you to deal with your weight issues and may make you feel better about yourself, in the long run you are denying the opportunity to accept control over your weight. Knowing that you <u>can</u> control your weight – that you <u>can</u> be slim and healthy – is a crucial step to take before starting to change your lifestyle. Slim people are very much in control of their weight and that is *not because* they are slim – it is *why* they are slim.

You <u>are</u> in control of your weight; do not let it control you

You may have felt like you have been trapped with weight issues, caused by a slow metabolism, or big bones, or genetics, or there may have been another justification that has not been mentioned here. You are not trapped, you can set yourself free. If we try to convince ourselves that we cannot change, we will not change. This is why you have to remove all these FALSE justifications, as then there will be nothing to stop you from moving on to thinking like a slim person. You will no longer have to justify your weight because you have accepted your weight and accepted that you can change it if you choose to. Weight loss will be much easier when there are no justifications to hold you back.

Once the comfort of these false justifications has gone, there may still be a tendency to try and defend, saying, "yes, but it's still not my fault that I'm overweight!" This is a natural reaction. Remember that nobody has the right to blame you, or judge you about your weight. However, if you have decided that you want to lose weight, it is up to you to say, "I am in CONTROL of my weight, I can change it if I CHOOSE to". Bear in mind that slim people have CHOSEN to be slim and you can too.

If you are still convinced that you really do not have a choice to control your weight, unfortunately you may find yourself stuck. It may be difficult to change an attitude which has been with you for such a long time, and it takes a lot of confidence. Sometimes this can be quite scary, and it can almost seem better to be trapped in a situation which you don't like, but which you know is safe, rather than be brave and take control and change. We can often seek reassurances from our friends and families, who then try to help us with our justifications, to make us feel better. This will only act to keep us where we are and create a vicious cycle which can be very tough to break out of.

If you are not happy with your current weight, then you have absolutely nothing to lose by changing your attitude towards it (except a little bit of weight!).

In order to regain control of your weight, you must stop justifying it. You must just accept it, and accept that you have the power to change it. You can then move on to weight loss if you choose to. Does that feel good? It should do.

> ### False justifications take away your ability to control your weight; remove them to <u>regain</u> the control

We do not need to defend our weight

Being overly defensive about our weight can be just as destructive as using false justifications. Defensive statements are used in an attempt to protect ourselves, when we feel that we are being judged on our weight (which we shouldn't be). We rebel against the perceived judgement – however it is not empowering for us, as how can we feel in control of a situation which we don't admit exists!

In the next panel are some examples of defensive statements, which we have all heard at one time or another.

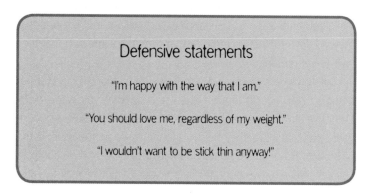

Defensive statements

"I'm happy with the way that I am."

"You should love me, regardless of my weight."

"I wouldn't want to be stick thin anyway!"

If you are happy exactly the way that you are, then congratulations, you have achieved what most people (slim or otherwise) will never truly achieve. However, if you are reading this book, you may not be as happy with your weight as you would like everyone else to think! There is no harm in that; it is a perfectly natural reaction to try and defend yourself when you are at risk from being upset.

As for the second statement, yes, your partner, family and friends should love you for who you are and not what weight you are, but this is an underhand tactic on your part to avoid the real issue. Just because somebody raised concerns about your health and well-being, doesn't mean that they do not love you. By all means, seriously consider the future of your relationship with someone who is giving you an ultimatum of, "lose weight or lose me", but be honest with yourself; has this ever actually happened? If your partner, or someone in your family, is worried about you, and worried about your weight, then you owe it to them to take their concerns seriously. It probably took a lot of courage in the first place to approach the topic and the fact that they are worried shows that they love you. Concerns over somebody's weight are not limited to the way they look. There are several health issues associated with being overweight and it is only natural that those around you may want to warn you, if you are in danger of suffering any ill effects. There may be a real opportunity here to gain the support of loved ones while you embrace your new approach to weight loss. I'm sure that they will love the new slimmer you, exactly the same way that they love you at present.

Defensive behaviour is not good for your relationships and is not going to help you to lose weight, if that is what you want to do. Defensive statements aren't so much about handing over control of your weight; however they are denying that there are real issues in the first place. Never underestimate how difficult it is to fully admit to yourself that you have responsibility for your weight. Be realistic – it is always important to know what the 'problems' are before moving on to finding solutions.

In the treatment of addictions, it is important for people to first admit they are addicted. In order to regain control of your weight, it is first important to accept responsibility for your weight. Again, I do not mean to imply that you should be blaming yourself, or anybody else, just accept that you have the power to change your weight and move on.

You do not have to defend your weight, just accept it

Clare

Over the course of a couple of years, Clare developed a tendency to overeat. She always seemed to be hungry and therefore felt that she needed to eat a lot at each meal. She would eat chocolate or a muffin mid-morning, a large lunch, and usually a large dinner too. On the evenings that she socialised she found that she would always need to eat again before she went to bed – sometimes this was a light snack, but often it was pizza, or a kebab. When she stayed in, she would snack on crisps or sweets. She compensated for this by walking to work and she also enjoyed the odd yoga class.

Although she had gone from a size 12 to a size 16 in two years, to her friends and family it seemed that Clare was very content with her weight. However, Clare did not like being overweight. She did not want to admit this, and so she didn't discuss it with anyone. Whenever any conversations came around to the subject of dieting, or weight, she would get very defensive. Eventually Clare confided to a friend that she did want to lose weight. At first she felt like she was being judged, and that she had somehow admitted defeat, but after a while she realised that she could just accept the fact that she was overweight and work towards changing it.

Clare lost weight initially by reducing her portion sizes, while still eating enough to satisfy her hunger. She also changed some of her unhealthy snacks for some healthier alternatives. Clare is now a size 14 and is starting to introduce more exercise into her routine in order to lose some more weight. More importantly than weight loss though, Clare has accepted her weight, has accepted that she can change it and has stopped feeling like she needs to justify or defend herself.

We are focusing here on helping <u>you</u> to feel in control of your weight, without feeling the need to justify or to defend yourself. Although this will be quite personal for you, there is nothing wrong with gaining the support of your friends and family, as long as they do not undermine your ability to control your own lifestyle. It is especially important that you do not let others, who wish to hold onto their own justifications and defensive behaviours, influence you. Remember the reasons why they still need to justify and defend – they are not in control and will remain stuck with a feeling of helplessness. No doubt, they will begin to come around when they notice the positive influence that being in control is having on your weight! These good effects may also spill over into other areas of your life, improving your confidence and your self-esteem.

Avoid everyday excuses

Once you can recognise the defensive and blaming attitudes that may have been holding you back, you can begin to accept your weight. You can then move forward – without blame and without judgement. You can choose to be slim, and look at your lifestyle to see what you want to change or prioritise, to achieve your ultimate goal.

The next hurdle to overcome is to recognise how easy it is to let everyday excuses slow your progress. We are all guilty of this; if we make excuses to ourselves we are again removing control and the acceptance that our choices affect our weight. We can CHOOSE to do something or we can CHOOSE not to do something. Excuses tend to creep in when we are trying to deny that we have a choice. We can choose slim options, lead a slim lifestyle and be slim, or we can make ourselves feel like we are being 'forced' into an action that we cannot control.

In the next panel are some of the more common excuses that are used. You could probably add a few more of your own, and excuses are not limited to people who have weight issues. I have used several of these myself in the past to justify my actions. (I am still working on not making excuses; it is a very hard habit to get out of!) Take a moment to think about the excuses that you might be using regularly.

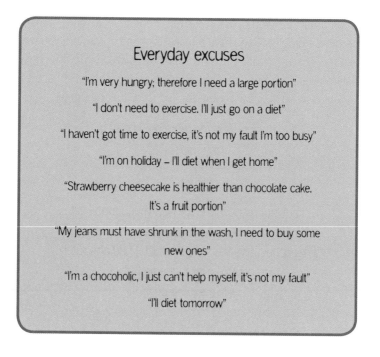

Everyday excuses

"I'm very hungry; therefore I need a large portion"

"I don't need to exercise. I'll just go on a diet"

"I haven't got time to exercise, it's not my fault I'm too busy"

"I'm on holiday – I'll diet when I get home"

"Strawberry cheesecake is healthier than chocolate cake. It's a fruit portion"

"My jeans must have shrunk in the wash, I need to buy some new ones"

"I'm a chocoholic, I just can't help myself, it's not my fault"

"I'll diet tomorrow"

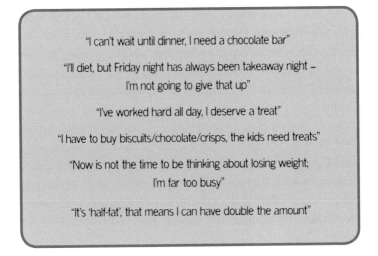

"I can't wait until dinner, I need a chocolate bar"

"I'll diet, but Friday night has always been takeaway night –
I'm not going to give that up"

"I've worked hard all day, I deserve a treat"

"I have to buy biscuits/chocolate/crisps, the kids need treats"

"Now is not the time to be thinking about losing weight;
I'm far too busy"

"It's 'half-fat', that means I can have double the amount"

Although everyone makes excuses from time to time, it only becomes a problem if you have actually managed to convince yourself that the excuse is valid. It is worth seriously considering every single statement and working out what exactly it is about each one that tries to deny that we have the control over our choice. For example;

"I'm <u>very</u> hungry; therefore I <u>need</u> a
large portion".

This statement could be rewritten as,

"I am 'not responsible' for how much food I eat
at my next meal. I will be <u>forced</u> to eat more than
I need, because the hunger, which I had absolutely
'no control' over in the first place,
will <u>make</u> me do it".

Now the second way of wording that excuse is very long-winded, but both statements are saying the same thing. You are trying to convince yourself that you are powerless to avoid a big meal, and that it is acceptable, because it's not really your fault.

Now let's look at the situation as it really is. It was effectively YOUR CHOICE to get too hungry, you were IN CONTROL over your hunger and could have CHOSEN to avoid getting too hungry (by having a healthy snack). Even if you had ignored the hunger until it was too late you could still CHOOSE what size meal you have. If you CHOOSE to have a normal meal, and you still feel hungry you can then CHOOSE to have a dessert, but the chances are you won't <u>need</u> a dessert to satisfy the hunger. Alternatively, you could CHOOSE to have a large meal. Do not excuse your decision, just make a straightforward set of choices and be in control.

Thinking situations through like this will make you much more aware that *your choices* are very important; there isn't anybody or anything that is 'forcing' you into situations that you cannot control. You can be in control of your weight, by being in control of situations like these. However, if you know that this sort of situation WILL cause you to choose to overeat, avoid it in the first place. Prioritise being slim over getting too hungry. I have learnt that I find it hard to make rational decisions when I am hungry (my family and friends have also noticed it), so I avoid getting too hungry in the first place. This leaves me able to CHOOSE what I want to eat, and not feel like I have been *forced* into overeating.

Let's try another common excuse;

> "I'll diet, but Friday night has always been takeaway
> night – I'm not going to give that up"

could be rewritten,

> "I'm going to have to really 'suffer' in order to
> lose weight. I won't enjoy the process at all;
> in fact I'm so hard done by that I 'need' to reward
> myself with a treat for all the suffering that
> I'm going through."

Okay, it's probably a little melodramatic, but can you see the victim card being played here? Saying "I deserve" is trying to justify ourselves again. This kind of thinking occurs when we have let a diet control us. Instead of feeling like we are in control, we have passed the control over to the diet. We then rebel against the 'evil diet', which is making us miserable, and we treat ourselves. Personally, I do not like diets for this very reason. However if you CHOOSE to go on a diet, and then CHOOSE to sabotage it with a curry every Friday night then you need to accept that it was your CHOICE to do so.

Now, I'm not telling you that you can't have a curry on a Friday night (if I was I would be taking the control away from you), however *you* must CHOOSE whether, or not, you have a curry on a Friday night rather than feel like you can't help it, or that you deserve it. You also must admit that, in the above situation, you have actually made having a curry on a Friday night a priority over losing weight on the diet. That's fine, you are not being blamed or judged for that, but it's important to accept that it was your CHOICE.

All the excuses listed reduce our ability to make a rational CHOICE by either falsely justifying a decision ("I <u>have</u> to buy chocolate, the kids <u>need</u> their treats"), defending a decision ("I'll diet when I <u>need</u> to; at the moment I'm having fun"), undermining our ability to decide rationally ("I'm a chocoholic, I just <u>can't help</u> myself, it's <u>not my fault</u>") or just plain kidding ourselves ("It's half-fat, I can have double the amount").

It is very interesting, why we try to trick ourselves into feeling like we have no control. Humans are programmed to eat and we need to eat otherwise we will die. However there is a lot more nice food around than we could ever need. At the same time humans have also been given the ability to think ahead and make rational decisions, so saying that we are programmed to eat and therefore we can't control ourselves is another false justification. Therefore the NEED to eat is in conflict with the NEED to control ourselves, otherwise we will eat far too much (which would be just as detrimental to our health as not eating enough). With all this nice food available, we know that we don't always *want* to make the 'right' choices (and it is difficult), so by denying that we have the CHOICE, we can enjoy what we want to without feeling guilty. We often do not have the confidence to deliberately make the 'wrong' choice, neither do we want to be seen to be making the 'wrong' choice – so we deny that the choice ever really existed.

Unfortunately we have got so good at making excuses that we really have convinced ourselves. As a result, we often feel forced into making 'naughty' choices AND we feel guilty about them, so we don't even enjoy them. Can you remember the last time that you did this? We will only ever be able to let go of the guilt and confidently enjoy our naughty choices when we are in control of ALL of our choices.

Learn to separate "I NEED" from "I WANT"

Self-esteem

There are lots of people for whom being a little bit overweight is something that they feel they need to get around to dealing with at some point, but it doesn't really have an impact on how they feel about themselves. They are not in despair about their weight and do not feel out of control. These people should find it very easy to abandon any justifications and excuses, and begin to change their lifestyles and lose weight, if that is what they choose to do. However, for others, excess weight can have a huge impact on self-esteem.

Instead of just not liking 'the weight', we often don't like ourselves, because of the weight, and feel very fed up. Everybody has days where they don't feel like they look their best and this affects the way that they feel. Take a step back and think, does the way that you look have a <u>huge</u> impact on the way that you feel? If so, it is an indication that you are suffering with low self-esteem. Redirecting all the negativity that comes from 'the weight' onto ourselves is not good. Low self-esteem can make you feel very helpless about your weight, making you feel less and less in control which can often lead to gaining even more weight.

It is not just 'the weight' that is responsible for low self-esteem, it is the feeling of being powerless over the weight. This is another way that dieting will fail in the long run. We wrongly assume that we will begin to feel much better about ourselves once we have lost some weight; however, we have not tackled the real cause of the low self-esteem, which is the feeling of helplessness. The diet gives us power over the weight temporarily, but as soon as the diet finishes, this feeling will disappear. Even if the diet is a success and you manage to lose some weight, you will not have learnt how to properly control YOUR weight in a way that suits YOU. You <u>can</u> regain the control which will stop you from feeling helpless about your weight. In turn this should help boost your self-esteem.

Start thinking 'slim'

The first step to becoming a slim person is to start thinking like a slim person. Regain control of your lifestyle and your weight by moving away from apportioning blame, or being defensive. Slim people have *chosen* to be slim, they have a *ccepted responsibility* for their weight and *chosen* to *control* it. The only advantage a slim person has over some-one who is overweight is that they have learnt, or were taught this, earlier on.

The change in attitude may not happen immediately. This is because attitudes are like habits; we are so used to them that they 'just happen' and often we do not question or challenge them. Just like the lifestyle habits that were making us gain weight need to change, so does the attitude that we are not in control of our weight.

Thinking like a slim person is just as important as acting like a slim person

Along with the new found 'control' will come the confidence to make 'slim' choices. The knowledge that all your choices have been made without justifications or denials, will help to overcome the guilt habit that lots of people have developed. Knowing that you are in control will diminish guilt. If you make a decision, have the confidence to follow it through without feeling guilty. If you CHOOSE to do some-thing then do it and enjoy it. DO NOT feel guilty.

So to recap, the following things will hold you back from weight loss and will not improve your self-confidence or your self-esteem:

- justifying why you are overweight by blaming something out of your control,

- being overly defensive about your weight or pretending that you are happy with it when you are not (not many people are happy with their weight, including lots of slim people),

- making excuses that attempt to remove the responsibility from yourself,

- feeling guilty about eating something after making a choice to do so.

By not needing to justify or defend, and not feeling guilty or making excuses, you will be taking a lot of pressure off yourself. There should be a real sense of freedom in being able to choose without feeling guilty. Be yourself, accept your weight, whatever it is and lose weight if you choose to. It's as simple as you make it!

'Think slim'

Look at the bigger picture

One of the biggest issues surrounding weight control is the lack of association between cause and effect. Everybody knows that if you eat high fat foods, you will be more prone to weight gain. Unfortunately, we can eat a lot of the 'wrong' type of food before any negative effect begins to show up around our waistlines. That makes it very difficult to identify exactly what it is that we are doing to cause the weight gain. We can also get so used to our habits that we do not notice what we do, therefore we don't really understand why we are carrying excess weight. Making a few small healthy changes to your lifestyle may not make you feel like you are making any serious progress. Rest assured that this is the best approach to maintainable weight loss. Every small step towards a healthy lifestyle adds up towards achieving a healthy weight.

The time delay between changing your lifestyle and your weight altering to catch up can also catch us out. What if our job changes and we find ourselves relying on convenience foods a bit more, and eating out a lot, as a mechanism to cope with the demands of the job? This is aside from the fact that the new job appears to have removed 'being slim' from the priorities list! At the end of week one, it is unlikely that we have noticed any weight gain. In fact, it may be a long time until any change would become noticeable. Then there is the risk that we will not associate the change in weight with the change in lifestyle (as, by that point, our new lifestyle has become normal). We can feel as if we have 'suddenly' put the weight on despite the fact that we have not been living like a slim person for weeks, or even months. This is because it is difficult to associate your weight with your whole lifestyle over a period of time. Your weight will eventually catch up to reflect your lifestyle.

A similar thing occurs with drinking to excess, but the association is much clearer, as the timescale is much shorter. Have you ever had too much alcohol, knowing full well you will get a hangover and then regretted it the following morning? I know I have.

If, for example, three drinks was my personal limit – by that I mean the maximum that I could drink, without causing a hangover – and I were to have four, or five drinks one evening, I would have a hangover in the morning. By the time I am feeling the effects, it is too late to prevent, or undo the damage. The association between cause and effect is very clear yet many people, myself included, still overindulge. We choose to forget the association. No doubt if I developed a hangover instantaneously when I had gone over my limit, I would never finish the third drink, let alone start the fourth!

We sometimes choose to forget the association between overeating, or eating the wrong foods, and putting weight on. Like the hangover example, if we were to instantaneously put on a stone, or go up a dress size after eating a takeaway meal, we probably would never even touch it (just like the fourth drink). Fortunately we do not gain excess weight in this way, otherwise the clothes that we wore at the beginning of the evening would not fit us at the end! Instead our body deals with the energy that it requires and stores the rest as fat. This build up of excess fat can be such a gradual process that it is very difficult to notice. The same goes for losing weight. We can 'diet' all week and not seem to get anywhere. It then feels like there is no point in carrying on with the diet. At our lowest points we can convince ourselves that there is no difference between 'being good' all week and 'being bad' therefore we may as well take the latter option as we tend to enjoy that a little bit more.

How does 'thinking slim' help?

Slim people have a better grasp of the association concept. It goes deeper than 'knowing' that high fat foods can make you fat. It is knowing it, and being able to factor that into their decision making, without letting justifications or excuses get in the way. It is not about self-denial, it is about deciding that the long-term consequences of a particular action are not worth the short-term benefits. This may seem difficult at first; however as your 'slim choices' start to pay off and you start to lose weight, it will become easier to make these decisions. It is the everyday decisions about food and exercise that all add up to a big impact on your weight. This is not an all-or-nothing approach, there is no requirement to make slim choices all of the time. However, the more slim choices you make, the more impressive your weight loss will be.

Old justifications and excuses could have previously been holding you back, by deliberately adding false reasoning to your decision making. This resulted in you fighting against yourself, or the diet, instead of looking at the bigger picture of wanting to be slim. To be slim, you must prioritise being slim, and make decisions which reflect that. When you are thinking like a slim person, you are aware of your actions. Instead of not noticing what you are eating, or drinking, you can consciously decide to do something, rather than doing it automatically.

Thinking like a slim person simplifies decision making. Imagine you are at a restaurant for dinner. You have already eaten dinner, maybe even a starter beforehand. The decision you now have to make is, "do I have dessert?" Previously, you may not even have asked yourself that question, and just automatically ordered a dessert.

Let's try and answer that question, firstly whilst thinking like a slim person, with being slim as a priority. We will then look at making that decision using the old way of thinking.

Situation: Dinner at a restaurant
Decision: Should I have the dessert?

Thinking like a slim person

Pros

"It looks like it will taste nice"

Cons

"If I eat too much fattening food, I will put on weight"

Old way of thinking

Pros

"It looks like it will taste nice"

"Everyone else is having some"

"I've been good all week, I deserve it"

"I've had a big dinner, dessert won't make any difference"

Cons

"If I eat too much fattening food, I will put on weight"

Thinking like a slim person, you have balance in your pros and cons list. You can choose between enjoying your dessert, because it tastes nice, and not having the dessert, because of the effect that it may have on your weight. Of course, I am not saying that one dessert will make you fat; however regularly eating fatty foods, or overeating in general without doing sufficient exercise, will cause weight gain. The decision can be made taking into account your whole lifestyle, with balance and moderation being the key. If the meal that preceded desert was very light and healthy, or you have been compensating all week, then that can be taken into consideration when deciding. To have the dessert, or not to have the dessert? It is your choice.

Compare this to the old way of thinking. Immediately we can see that by simply adding more reasons to the pros list, we have engineered it so that there are more pros than cons. This makes it more difficult to make a logical decision as we have thrown in illogical reasoning.

Does it really matter if everybody else is having dessert? Why does that mean that you have to follow the crowd? If you have had a big dinner then surely that is even more of a reason to pass on dessert if your aim is to be slim? As for deserving it, what exactly have you done to specifically deserve it? All of these reasons are false justifications, which you may previously have subconsciously added to your pros list to make it outweigh the cons. This will make it seem like a really big sacrifice to go without dessert – the self-denial feels huge, because you have put far too much importance on having the dessert.

This can even lead to the classic situation of having eaten too much for dinner, then having a dessert that you couldn't really manage. You then feel guilty and uncomfortably full. Have you ever felt like you can't move after dinner, except maybe to loosen your belt? Incidentally, I do this every year at Christmas dinner! I don't feel guilty about it, as it is not a holiday from 'being slim', just an indulgence which I factor in and therefore easily compensate for. I put overdoing it during Christmas dinner as a higher priority than being slim temporarily, and I really enjoy it. Inevitably, I always feel very uncomfortable afterwards, but it helps remind me that, in general, I much prefer to avoid overeating, although I can cope with it once a year.

Last Christmas morning, my husband and I went for a walk. It was a lovely cold, but sunny day and lots of other people were also out and about for some fresh air. We were only out for about 30 minutes but we saw four or five joggers. We were very impressed, as it takes a lot of effort to get out for a run on such a cold day, especially a holiday. I bet that these fit, healthy and slim people did not feel in the slightest bit guilty about tucking into a big dinner.

So how does this relate to you trying to decide whether or not to have a dessert? Remember in this scenario you have already enjoyed your dinner, possibly even a starter before that. So you are not starving yourself. The chances are that you don't require the dessert in order to survive, or even to just to feel comfortably full. You may even be feeling pretty full already. The decision is based purely on indulgence and has nothing to do with hunger or 'needing' to eat. This is where the lifestyle balance comes into it. If we ate a three course meal on our birthdays or at Christmas for example, it would not affect our weight over the year in the slightest. On the other hand, if we were to eat a three course meal twice a week, then we would be very soon buying jeans in the next size up!

Let's go back to 'slim' thinking – we can see how weighing up the pros and cons can help us make the decision. If you thought that the dessert was going to taste absolutely wonderful, and therefore would be well worth the (cumulative) effect on your weight, the decision to have the dessert becomes easy and guilt-free. Examples of this would be, if it's your favourite dessert which is on offer or you don't have dessert often (or it's your birthday).

The pros and cons balance can also tip the other way when we are thinking like a slim person. What if we don't think the dessert will be worth the effect on our weight? Why waste a dessert opportunity if you don't actually really like what's on offer that much? In that case it is easy to decide that being slim is worth missing dessert for.

The difficult bit is the middle ground, where the dessert looks really nice AND we want to be slim. This is when your priorities are really tested. If 'being slim' is your priority, then CHOOSE not to have the dessert, or choose to have a smaller portion. Little things all add up. Initially, you will probably feel like you are missing out on the dessert, but there will be others! Being slim requires a lifestyle approach. That means you can have the occasional indulgence, but the key is balance and moderation. In return, you will have a nice slim body. You cannot have a nice slim body and eat whatever you want – nobody can.

It is what you do most of the time that has the biggest impact on your weight

If you choose not to have the dessert then remember that it was your <u>choice</u> to make being slim a <u>priority</u> over eating the dessert so be careful not to moan about it. If you do, you will probably find your resolve weakening when people try to make you feel better with their own justifications and excuses. If you do choose to eat it, do not feel guilty; in the same way if you choose not to eat it, do not feel like a victim. Learning this new habit of making silent 'slim' decisions may take some getting used to. Don't worry if you find yourself being vocal about it initially and admitting to people that you are weighing up the pros and cons. Instead you can use it as an opportunity to observe other people's reactions to your change in behaviour. You may find that, if you choose to decline the offer of dessert, others try to encourage you to change your mind. This peer group pressure can be a powerful force, and it may startle you to discover that the people you know and love are holding you back from being slim by not respecting your decision.

We can see from the dessert example that thinking like a slim person allows you to better see the association between behaviour and consequence, as the consequence has not been overshadowed by the exaggerated importance of the behaviour. By being more aware of the associations, it is easier to see the benefits of choice. It is then not about self-denial; instead it is a choice of priorities, it is about seeing the bigger picture. That picture may be you in a size ten dress or on a beach in a skimpy bikini. If it helps, take a moment to picture yourself in your favourite shop trying on a pair of skinny jeans, and not wondering "does my bum look big in this?"

On other occasions, the bigger picture may be indulging in life's little pleasures, or if you are eating at a friend's house, not offending the host that has baked you a dessert! Be careful with that last one though, it could easily become a false justification.

To emphasize, this does <u>not</u> mean that you have to <u>always</u> choose to not have something fattening, or always choose the slim option. This is part of the whole lifestyle approach and it is your choice what you do. You can still enjoy your favourite foods (in moderation, of course), and have the odd indulgence whilst working towards your ultimate goal of being slim. If you can see the bigger picture and have a lifestyle approach to weight loss, then you can also apply the accumulation factor to decision making. Lots of 'slim' or healthy choices will, over time, add up to a big difference to your weight. Making lots of slim choices takes the pressure off each individual choice, allowing you to really enjoy saying, "yes!" to something every now and again. I'm sure that you will enjoy getting to your eventual target much more if you do not feel like you are constantly depriving yourself along the way.

At first these decisions may seem hard and you may still always want to choose to have something, or always feel guilty even when you are trying not to. Like anything else though, it is just a case of getting into the habit of making decisions. Over time you will really get to know your body – it may sound strange – but you will get to the stage where you can 'feel' whether you can indulge or not. Instead of sitting there and having to think about your choices, it will become automatic; you will instinctively know whether the indulgence can be easily compensated for or not. You will then be that slim person, who can choose to not have something with no fuss, or choose to have it without guilt. At that point, when you are truly thinking like a slim person, you will have banished any feelings of guilt or self-denial forever.

The knowledge that something is high in fat will not help you to not eat it, if you feel that you have an uncontrollable urge to eat it. All the knowledge will do is give you something to feel guilty about once you have actually eaten it. However, if the attitude is right and we are thinking like a slim person, then we will have fewer uncontrollable urges, only very controllable 'wants'. If we know that our lifestyle is balanced and healthy most of the time, then we can make the decision to have something – for example, a chocolate bar – and not feel guilty. Alternatively, we can decide not to have the chocolate bar, and not feel like we have deprived ourselves, as there are other rewards, such as being one step closer to a slim figure. This is a million miles away from "I deserve," or "I can't help myself," or "I'm not allowed." Once you have conquered 'thinking slim', you are truly ready to 'act slim'!

'Act Slim'

What do I need to do?

Hopefully you have been pleasantly surprised to discover that slim people do not have any natural advantage, but have different attitudes and habits that keep them slim. Learning the *Thin Secrets* should have convinced you that taking control will make a world of difference to your weight. By now I suspect that you are chomping at the bit to start trying out new slim ways as part of a new slim lifestyle. This chapter is where you can learn how to apply the *Thin Secrets* to effectively lose weight. The best part is that there is no dieting involved. Ever!

The 'dieters' may find it very frustrating to not have a clear set of eating rules that they can photocopy and attach to the fridge door with a magnet. It may seem to be very alien not to have calorie charts, or food diaries to fill in daily. This book is about letting you feel in control of your weight, and being ready to change your lifestyle in order to lose weight. This is not about learning 'the rules'. Rules take away our control and choice. However, we can work within some general guidelines. The best way to ensure that we achieve a healthy weight is to aim for a healthy lifestyle. Don't worry, this does not mean eating nothing but fruit and going for a run at 6am every morning. A healthy lifestyle and weight balance is about finding things that you like that are also good for you.

We have seen how 'thinking slim' can help us to make more slim decisions, now we need to apply those in our lives, in order to lose weight. Knowing what is good for our health and what is not so good helps us to make more slim choices; however, there is no need to count calories, or become obsessed with food like we might on a diet.

Your routines and habits are very personal to you, and therefore it is difficult to prescribe a set of changes to make. In general, slim people, as well as being in control of their choices, and making more slim choices than not, also have compensation mechanisms which they use to stay slim. By this I mean that a binge, or indulgence may be followed by an extra effort to get back on track in the following days, with careful eating or some extra exercise. However, when you are trying to lose weight, you may choose to limit the indulgences and extend the compensation periods for a while, in order to see results more quickly. This still means that you can (choose to) have the occasional treat, and really enjoy it. However, the treats may need to be a little bit more modest than they will be once you have reached a weight you are happy with. Basically, the more effort that you put in, the more that you will get out of it.

Maintaining any particular weight is much easier than losing weight. However it is still important to put effort into weight maintenance. So if you do have those periods where you seem to be not making any progress, as long as you are maintaining your weight and not putting any on, then you know that you have the balance right for your present lifestyle. These periods are very useful as they allow you to look closely at the cause/effect balance. All that is required to start losing weight is to tip the balance. Introduce some more small changes and make more slim choices, including more exercise. Your long term goal should be weight maintenance, once you have achieved your slim body. With dieting, weight maintenance is seen as failure – it is not.

If you feel like a member of the life-long diet club, you may consider yourself as something of an expert in the calorific values and fat contents of certain foods. This will work to your advantage, when making slim choices. You do not, however, have to be a nutritionist, or a doctor to know that generally cutting down on fats, reducing overall calorie intake and doing more exercise is the route to weight loss. This is the energy balance that we discussed earlier, and short of drastic surgery, we can't cheat it. It is as much a part of life as death or taxes. There is no way round it, but by accepting it, we can move on to finding the easiest and most enjoyable way to work the system.

Knowing how the energy balance works is the easy bit, knowing what you should be eating and drinking as part of a healthy diet is also easy. It's putting it into practice that is hard. That is what this book is about.

Avoid hunger

I have found that it is important to not let myself get too hungry. It is a habit that I have had to work at changing. Hunger is probably my biggest motivator for overeating, as I am sure it is for a lot of people. If you get very hungry you may find it extremely difficult to make slim choices.

If we did not eat, we would eventually die. We need food to survive, but we also enjoy food and go and seek it out if we haven't had any for a while. We recognise this as hunger. Our instinct to eat may have remained the same for generations, but the availability and the quality of the food has changed. Whereby our early ancestors spent their days hunting and gathering for food, we can have it delivered, pre-cooked to our doors. When it comes to the quality of the food, we are very lucky to have a wide variety of tastes and flavours available to us, but we have also developed a fondness for very energy-dense foods. On top of all this, our bodies are very efficient at storing up any excess energy as fat, which is then available to us in periods of starvation. Often we are not using up all the energy that we gain from our food, and our very efficient energy storage systems go into overdrive converting the excess into fat (for our own benefit – of course).

In modern day society, the food will always be in plentiful supply. It will never be necessary for us to stock-up for a long, cold, harsh winter where the food will be scarce. Fortunately, we don't have to suffer long periods of starvation, we only have to 'survive' until the next meal (or overnight until breakfast), so we rarely have an opportunity to use up our fat supplies, but we continue to add to them.

This is why it requires effort to remain slim. We are fighting against natural urges to stockpile in times of plenty. It would be so much easier to just let nature take its course and eat. After all, that is what we are programmed to do! I am not trying to provide a false justification for overeating, as although it would be easier to give in to all the urges, inevitably we would become very fat. We all know that gaining too much extra fat will damage our health. Therefore an evolutionary mechanism designed to keep a species alive has become an enemy to our health, unless we can keep it under control. This conflict helps to explain why we have an obesity epidemic on our hands.

Regardless of the health implications of being obese, most people do not actually want to be overweight. This is because it affects the way they look, and the way that they feel about themselves. There are lots of very good reasons, which help us understand that although we have a natural tendency to eat more than we require, it is important not to act on it all of the time. Slim people still feel the urges; they just do not act on them all the time.

The urge to eat is still an important instinct; we still need to feel hunger. If we did not have an instinctive drive to eat, then we would die much more quickly from starvation than we would by going the other way and developing obesity-linked disorders. Despite the urges though, most people do not want to be left with a large store of excess body fat.

To suggest that the best way to become slim is to ignore your hunger urges is pretty much going against nature itself. If you are hungry, eat. If you do not eat when you are hungry then you may go on to crave more energy-dense foods to satisfy a more intense hunger. Hunger is not bad for you. It is your body's way of letting you know that you want to be fed. Don't allow hunger to cloud your choice though. 'Hunger' can convince you that you can eat a lot more than you need. 'Hunger' may make you feel like you NEED to have a certain type of food. Your logical brain may have to override your stomach on that one, and it is difficult for the brain to win when it is fighting a hungry stomach! Hunger has probably got in the way of many a dieter's good intentions and it can be a very strong motivator.

If you find that it is tough for you to make a slim choice when you are hungry (I do) then plan for it. Either don't let yourself get overly hungry (it's an unpleasant feeling anyway) or plan in advance what you are going to eat even before you get hungry. That way your decision is much more likely to be a well-balanced meal, or a sensible portion size. What you will be doing is making 'being slim' a priority and not putting yourself into situations where in the past you may have over-eaten, or eaten unhealthily.

If hunger causes you to overeat, avoid getting too hungry

When you are hungry it is very easy for you to trick yourself into thinking that your body needs something specific, that something plain, or healthy will not do. This is a psychological craving, not a biological one. A hamburger may satisfy a psychological craving much better then it satisfies nutritionally! However, from a survival point of view a sandwich will probably do! When you are hungry you need to eat. However, try to choose healthy options and recognise that cravings are often hunger in a clever disguise.

We live in a society which doesn't like hunger; there is always somewhere that you can pick up a snack or meal. Unfortunately, healthy snacks are not as widely available as unhealthy ones. It is very easy to buy a chocolate bar, or a bag of crisps at newsagents, vending machines and service stations. It is less easy to get hold of healthier snacks, and it is most likely cheaper to buy a burger from a fast food restaurant than it is to buy a low-fat sandwich from a supermarket.

If you often get hungry and feel like you have no choice other than to buy an unhealthy snack when you are out, or travelling, why not go back to basics and take snacks, or even packed lunches out with you? Even just having a banana or some biscuits with you may save you from getting so hungry that you 'need' to have a pasty or a king-size chocolate bar just to get you through. Yes, it requires a bit of forward planning, but all the little things add up.

Drink plenty of water

There is a theory that being dehydrated can cause false feelings of hunger. This could lead to eating to satisfy the 'hunger' instead of drinking to satisfy the thirst. To avoid dehydration it is recommended that we all drink eight glasses of water a day (more if you are exercising). Have a drink before or whilst you eat, and if you have alcohol with a meal consider having a soft-drink as well. Although it may be worth having a drink when you feel hungry, just in case the feelings are caused by thirst, the drawback is that you may actually need to eat and that delaying may cause you to get too hungry. This could result in overeating. Like everything, it is up to you to find out what it is that works best for you.

Replace 'bad' habits with 'good' habits

It is important that you become very aware of what it is you do. Don't just get on with your normal routine, having the same breakfast, buying a chocolate bar with your magazine, going for lunch at the same place without taking a step back. If you want to, write down what you eat and drink on a daily basis. It might surprise you, it may not. See where you can make changes, even if all you can do one day is not have mayonnaise on your sandwich at lunchtime – that will add up, along with the other things that you do on other days.

Think about your weekly routine, and where you can fit exercise in. You may be very busy at the start of the week, but less busy towards the weekend. Does this mean that you should try and fit in exercise later in the week, or will it be harder to motivate yourself when you are less busy? It may be better to squeeze it into an already tight schedule earlier in the week. It is up to you to prioritise.

Good habits may be fairly easy to introduce into your routine, in order to help you reach your goal of being slim and healthy. Maybe you could start eating more fruit and vegetables every day, or start having breakfast, if you didn't already do so. Eating an apple instead of a biscuit may require less effort than putting on comfortable shoes and going for a walk, but every little thing that you do will add up.

Begin to identify and let go of bad habits. They have become habits because we feel comfortable with them. We like them and we may be reluctant to change. However, they may be preventing us from losing weight, or worse, causing us to gain weight.

Some examples of bad habits include:

- snacking unhealthily,
- having lots of fizzy drinks,
- eating large portions,
- eating fatty food regularly,
- having sugar in tea/coffee,
- having cheese as an extra on meals,

- driving instead of walking,

- eating lots of food high in sugar,

- never doing any exercise,

- having regular takeaway meals,

- drinking alcohol to excess,

- skipping meals and snacking instead.

Not only do the habits in the above list make us gain weight, but they can also be detrimental to our health. Many disorders can be directly linked to some of these bad habits, including type II diabetes, tooth decay, high cholesterol and heart disease. Obesity has also been linked to an increased risk of developing certain cancers. It is worth stopping to think about this for a few moments. Altering your diet can drastically improve your health and your life expectancy. Not only could you potentially live longer, but you could spend that time having fewer worries about your health. In many cases the long-term damage that has been caused by an unhealthy diet, cannot be fixed with pills or operations. You only have one life, is it not worth living to the full by being as healthy as you can easily be?

Once you have identified your particular bad habits, then it is time for you to work out your strategy for each. You may want to tackle them one at a time, or you may want to go for an all-or-nothing approach. The more drastic the lifestyle change, the more drastic the weight loss will be, but the harder it will be to stick with. Remember that your new lifestyle has to be something that you enjoy and that you can maintain.

The best thing about the lifestyle approach is that the smallest, simplest habits can often have the biggest impact. Do you buy your own lunch everyday? You can easily save money and be healthier by taking your own sandwiches instead.

If you are used to eating canteen food, or grabbing fast-food, then switching to healthy home-made sandwiches will quickly have an effect on your weight. Taking the extra time in the morning to prepare them will probably be a hassle at first, but it will soon become part of your routine and you won't notice it. You may even end up saving time that would have been spent buying food during the day. That allows you more time to relax, or even fit in a short walk at lunchtime. The money that you save will also soon add up.

If you often get hungry mid-afternoon, then pack an extra sandwich as a healthy snack. Obviously, if you don't get hungry then you don't need to eat it!

The obvious place to start is to get rid of, or cut down on, the things you won't miss too much. If you drink cola because you prefer it to water, then it may seem like a hardship to go back to water. However, does it make any difference to you whether you drink cola or the diet alternative? How about blackcurrant juice, or orange squash instead? If you change the things that you won't miss anyway you can potentially make a huge difference to your lifestyle, and therefore your weight, with very little effort.

The other approach is to change whatever it is that will make the biggest difference first. If one of your bad habits is actually eating too much, then cutting down on portion sizes will have a huge impact on your weight, regardless of whether you change the type of food that you eat or not.

Replacing a 'bad' habit with a 'good' habit may be easier than giving something up all together. For example, switching from butter to low-fat spread is a small change which over time can make a big difference, and won't actually take very long to get used to.

There are plenty of other habits which you will be able to change in your daily routine. This is maybe where your slim friends could help you out. Find out what other people do to make those little compensations which add up to the difference between maintaining a slim figure, and gaining weight.

At the end of the day, it is up to you to find a nice balance in your lifestyle between being healthy and slim, and enjoyment. Losing weight and staying slim requires effort but it doesn't have to be miserable, unless of course you choose to be miserable about it! If being slim is a priority for you then you are not a victim of a diet; instead you are working for yourself, to achieve your own weight loss goals.

Here are some more suggestions of slim habits:

- have three healthy meals most days, to compensate for the occasional indulgent dinner,
- get into the habit of snacking healthily and always have a snack at easy access to avoid getting too hungry,
- make exercise part of your daily routine,
- get out of the habit of having dessert, so that it is a real treat whenever you do have it,

- don't get too hungry before going out for dinner, it will help you to choose the healthier option,

- vary your exercise so you don't get bored,

- avoid takeaways if you are trying to lose weight,

- gradually cut down on crisps, chocolate, and sweets until they become occasional treats,

- have a hobby which involves exercise, such as dance classes, horse-riding or walking the dog.

Being aware that your weight will always reflect your lifestyle allows you to formulate your own personalised 'Action Plan' for weight loss. This may be a very informal exercise of just deciding to make more of an effort to be healthier. Or you may choose to be extremely formal – reminiscent of the dieting days – and write out a detailed plan for yourself which you can attach to the fridge door. Do what ever it is that you need to do to make this work. You deserve to be slim and healthy! Unlike a diet plan, which is preconceived by somebody else, your Action Plan will be very personal to you, but it should be based on a whole lifestyle approach to weight loss. Although it may take some getting used to initially, in the long run it should be a lifestyle that will be easy for you to maintain. As a result your Action Plan will change. This is a good thing as it allows you to fine-tune your lifestyle until you discover what works for you.

It is your choice entirely what goes into your Action Plan (if you choose to have one at all). However, if you want to lose weight and be slim for life then it is your responsibility to take the next step and make it happen.

The following exercise may help you to produce your own person-alised Action Plan. It is entirely up to you whether you choose to do the exercise or whether you choose to devise your own strategy.

Bad habits: List everything that you do, or don't do, that may be considered an unhealthy, or weight-gaining, habit. It is important to include everything, even if you have absolutely no intention of changing it – the idea here is to recognise the link between cause and effect and understand what it is that may be contributing to excess weight. There is no need to feel guilty, or justify, or defend. Just write it all down.

Good habits: Now think about, and write down, all the good habits that you currently have, and add as many more that you can think of that would give you the healthiest lifestyle possible. This again can include things that you have no intention of doing any time soon (for example, training for a decathlon). However, it is important to realise how much you <u>could</u> be doing towards your goals, even if you choose not to.

Excuses: Have a think about your limitations. If you are car dependent, you cannot realistically jog to work in the morning. If you take these into account when you are making your plan, you have already removed all your valid excuses before you begin. Therefore it will be harder for excuses to impede your progress.

Action plan: Now look at both lists and choose how you would like to shape your new lifestyle. Select those unhealthy, weight-gaining habits that you would like to get out of and look at all the ways that you could introduce healthy habits. Be realistic; only include the things that you want to do, or that you are prepared to do in order to achieve your weight-loss goals and become healthier. This is your life and your list. You are the only one who can take responsibility for making it happen. Don't panic that you have to do everything at once; we will talk about timescales later on. For now, all that is important is that you have identified for yourself what you are prepared to do to become slim and healthy.

Eating out

Lots of people eat out on special occasions, and it can often be important not to feel like you are missing out, or that you are being restricted by a diet. As you are not on a diet, but choosing to be slim, there are several options available to you when eating out. You could choose to indulge and compensate the following day, or week. You could decide to have whatever you fancied for your main course, but not have, or cut back on a starter and dessert. Maybe you could share a course with somebody else? Alternatively you could look for a relatively healthy menu option that you will enjoy and that you will not need to compensate for! There is no requirement to overindulge whenever you eat out. However, there is also nothing wrong with the occasional indulgence!

If eating out is not just limited to special occasions for you, then there is all the more incentive to try some compromises. However, bear in mind that you are compromising between your desire to eat something fattening and your goal of being slim. You are not fighting against an evil diet, there is nothing forcing you.

A word of caution – avoid the buffet! Even the most resolute slim-thinking person can get carried away when faced with the prospect of unlimited nice food. The all-you-can-eat menu is a great idea in principle; in practice, it's like sending a group of students to a free bar event. Everyone inevitably consumes a lot more than is healthy! It may be worth not putting yourself in that situation for a while, rather than trying to be strong. As for buffets and snacks at parties (which you can't avoid), it might be worth serving yourself out a meal – one plateful of food – and then stopping, rather than grazing all evening. It will be easier to choose to stop eating when you can see that you haven't missed out. Alternatively, send somebody you trust to serve you a 'sensible' portion, so you don't ever get to see what is on offer. You will not be the only one trying to restrain yourself. There will be plenty of slim people in the room trying to do exactly the same thing!

The food on offer at buffets is usually quite fattening. This is deliberate as it is often the food that is the most popular. This is all the more reason to try and avoid overeating. Don't go hungry, as that would probably ruin your evening. You may feel it is necessary to eat healthily before you arrive and just have dessert (or a small taster) at the party, so that you don't feel like you have missed out.

Have a strategy for the buffet

Boredom and comfort eating

Social occasions can often revolve around food. Meals can be almost ritual-like, with certain foods eaten at certain times of the day, and 'special' food on special occasions. Therefore eating is more than just fulfilling hunger. It is about being sociable, relaxing, or treating yourself (as well as surviving).

Some foods, for example chocolate, release 'feel-good' chemicals in our brains, making eating more pleasurable. It's no wonder that we then choose to eat out of boredom, or to cheer ourselves up, without even being physically hungry. So-called 'comfort eating', can become a major habit, but that is all it is. If you are in the habit of eating for any reason other than being physically hungry, then you have a great opportunity to change something which is likely to have a drastic impact on your weight. Comfort eating may feel like it cannot be helped, but it can. All it needs is a strategy.

I'll use a fairly common example of 'chocolate addiction'. You may feel like you are addicted to chocolate, but it will only last while you are still eating chocolate! This sounds strange, but if you don't feed the habit, the cravings will go away.

Remember the earlier example of the smokers who were trying to quit? Those who want to stop smoking will do much better than those who feel that they ought to stop. The same goes for chocolate (although to a much lesser extent). If you associate your chocolate habit with your excess weight you may all of a sudden want to give it up.

Basically all you need to do in the first instance is <u>choose</u> not to eat chocolate. It boils down to a simple choice – do you want to feed your chocolate addiction, or do you want to maximise your chances of becoming slim? If you decide that you can't possibly go cold turkey on the chocolate, then cut down gradually. The week or two at first, when you really miss it, will be rewarded in the long run, with a slim figure – if that is what you choose.

Remember not to think of it as self-denial, but as an exchange between the short-term pleasure of the chocolate treat and the long-term pleasure of being slim. You might miss the chocolate, but the hard part will actually be breaking the habit, rather than going without. After the initial effort, you will no longer crave chocolate, and you will be out of the habit. Therefore the decision not to have chocolate will become much easier. Slim choices get easier, once you are in the habit of making them.

If you are used to having a bar of chocolate every single day, and you suddenly stopped, without replacing it, there would be a gaping hole where once there was chocolate. That hole needs to be filled, either with a healthier alternative snack, or with a distraction, such as a change of routine. So if you always had chocolate on your tea break at work, can you take your break in a different location? A change of routine may help you break the habit. If it is not practical to do that, how about replacing a chocolate bar with a hot chocolate drink or a different snack? It will be strange at first, but you'll get into the new habit soon enough – if you allow yourself to (and if you choose to do it)!

Chocolate addiction is not a serious condition!

There are, of course, two other ways to get the release of the feel-good chemicals, which don't involve food. The first is sex and the second is exercise, although you could argue that they are both just different forms of exercise! Both of these will also help with weight loss. It may not always be feasible to replace the chocolate with either of these (especially if you are at work at the time), but it's worth considering at other opportunities!

Believe it or not, it is possible to become addicted to exercise. This is not something that should worry most people and certainly shouldn't put anybody off. The buzz that you can get after exercising is a natural high and the more exercise you do, the more you will feel like doing – which is great!

Comfort eating, or eating out of boredom, is a very easy habit to get into and quite difficult to get out of. We may actually kid ourselves into thinking that we really are hungry. This is when priorities and careful decision making really come in to it. It may be necessary to force yourself to do something else, or change your routine to avoid the situations where you tend to eat unnecessarily. This will only be temporary, while you are trying to get out of habits. In addition, avoiding buying the foods that you are likely to eat out of boredom effectively forces you to eat healthily or nothing at all.

When I was growing up, I remember often wanting to eat in the evenings, after I had already had dinner. My mother would say, "there is always bread and jam if you are hungry". This seems quite old-fashioned now, but it worked. Nine times out of ten, I wouldn't eat the bread and jam on offer, I'd just go without. This made me realise that I actually wasn't particularly hungry, I just wanted to eat. If we had been allowed to help ourselves to biscuits and cakes as children, I'm sure nobody would ever have asked me if I had hollow legs!

I have tried to extend the same principle to my adult life. Often in the evenings, following a proper dinner, I still feel 'hungry' for something. If there was ice-cream or chocolate in the house, I would probably eat it. If I was offered bread and jam, or cereal, I would probably decline. Therefore, I rationalise that I'm not really hungry. Neither am I denying myself, as I have generally eaten three proper meals plus snacks throughout the day. I'm not physically hungry; I just have a case of evening 'munchies', which most of the time is psychological. The times when I find that I am actually genuinely hungry, I tend to have cereal, or toast as a filling low-fat snack (depending of course on the type of cereal you have and how much butter you put on your toast!).

Shop carefully

The time-tested rule has to be; do not shop on an empty stomach. Everyone knows that if you shop when hungry you will be much more tempted to buy anything and everything. It might be wise to go one step further in the initial stages of getting used to the new slimmer, healthier you, and take a very specific shopping list with you. Try and only buy what is on your list.

It may be useful to plan what you are going to eat for the rest of the week before you go shopping. Be realistic though, so you don't go over the top. Planning to eat nothing but lentils might backfire when you get sick of it mid-week and order a pizza.

Planning your meals before you shop should save you a bit of money, by avoiding the impulse buys. Don't be tempted by the buy-one-get-one-free offers. It may seem like good value at the time, but if it means you eat much more than you intended, then it is a bad investment. The big supermarkets have been criticised recently for putting more unhealthy foods on special offer to try to increase our spending. This is taking advantage of the temptation to buy sweet and fatty foods, although hopefully the trend is shifting towards the promotion of healthier alternatives as well.

Get into the habit of buying healthy food

Shopping itself is a habit. You probably go to the same places and buy the same types of food most of the time. Remember that the food that you choose to buy will be the food that you choose to eat later on. Therefore, it might be worth going shopping when you are focused on your goal of being slim, and while you are enthusiastic about making progress. For a while, avoid shopping if you are tired, or in a bad mood, or are likely to sabotage your weight loss efforts. It is only a temporary measure, until you get into new shopping habits of buying mainly healthy, 'slim' types of food, and avoiding the crisps and biscuits.

Clear the cupboards in preparation

So you have decided to change your lifestyle in order to lose weight. You are armed and ready with your shopping list and your list of good and bad habits is taped to the fridge door. What do you do with the food that is already in the house, that you will be trying so hard not to eat? It's a common problem. Do you leave it there and hope that you have enough will-power to avoid eating it? That is probably not a good plan; I don't really think there is anything to be gained from sitting and looking at something which you need to avoid eating most of the time.

Maybe you have considered eating it all quickly, to get it out of the way before you start to make your changes! Again, this is not an advisable strategy, just a feeble excuse for a major binge. If you feel the need to eat all the 'bad' foods before adopting a few lifestyle changes, then are you making being slim a priority for you? It is similar to the smoker's chant of, "I'll quit when I've finished the next packet". Make a clean break now; your enthusiasm is likely to be much higher at the very start of something new. It will be much easier to get rid of packet of chocolate digestives on day one when you are feeling motivated, then it will be to try and not eat them on day four, if they are still in the cupboard.

So what are you going to do with the food that you should be eating less of that is still in your kitchen cupboards? Could you give some of it away? Take it into work and share it out, perhaps? This will send a message out to your friends and colleagues that you are taking this lifestyle change seriously and you are inviting their support.

Don't forget you could always throw it away. This will be a real test of your determination to succeed. It's not ideal to waste food, but it is better to get rid of it than to store it on your body as excess fat! The concept of throwing food away will probably horrify some people as there are so many hungry people in the world. Unfortunately, the only person who is affected by whether or not you eat the food that is in your kitchen cupboards is you!

Clearing the cupboards of the foods that don't feature in your new lifestyle will make you feel like you are taking decisive action. You will be embracing an attitude change and it should make you feel positive, and confident that you are on the way to achieving your weight loss goals.

Get active

Obviously, I agree with the advice that you often see in magazines of parking the car a little bit further away and walking, or getting off the bus one stop earlier than usual. I even try to climb the stairs rather than taking the lift wherever possible. These are only small things, but they do add up when you take into account the accumulation factor. However, if you wish to lose weight and remain slim, you will have to do more than this. It is your choice entirely what you do (if anything at all), although I do feel that people often need that extra bit of encouragement when it comes to exercising.[3]

It wasn't until I started exercising regularly that I began to see the real benefits. If you do a variety of aerobic, resistance and stamina training, you will be well on the way to having a slim, toned body. This doesn't mean that you have to become a weight-lifter or a marathon runner, but do a variety of exercise. Combining an activity like swimming, cycling, brisk walking or jogging with something like circuit

3   If you are worried about whether or not you should be exercising then it is worth discussing it with your doctor first.

training or yoga, helps with general fitness, muscle tone and supple-ness. If only the diet part of your lifestyle changes, you will lose weight; however you can dramatically speed up the process by exercising at the same time. Over time, your fitness will improve, so you will get more out of each exercise session.

It doesn't matter if you never really done much exercise before, or haven't done any for a long time. Start slowly and carefully – it's never too late to start!

As your fitness improves you will feel better and have more energy. Although at first it may feel like too much effort to exercise, after a while you will really start to see the benefits in terms of weight loss and your energy levels. My husband had always told me that, for him, fitness was a vicious circle; the more you did, the more you enjoyed and felt like doing it. However once you stopped exercising regularly the harder it became to start each time. For a long time I didn't believe him – I became increasingly unconvinced after my first circuit training class! I kept at it though and over the following month my attitude changed dramatically. I had more energy and I even began to want to go for a run!

Doing <u>some</u> exercise is always better than doing none. Getting started may be hard but regular exercise is a good way to feel like you are actively working towards your weight loss goals, rather than just waiting for them to happen.

It is not necessary to go to the gym; if you find the idea a little scary, you are not alone. Surprisingly men are just as likely as women to find the gym intimidating.[4] Men are generally a bit more competitive than women and the 'competition' for men at gyms is often the body builder types. I would definitely find it intimidating to be lifting weights next to someone three times my size! Go to the gym if you want to, if not do something different, or go with a friend to get used to it before

4   From a survey carried out on students; 16% of men and 18% of women reported finding the gym intimidating.

you venture in on your own. Prioritise your aim of a slim, toned body over the potential embarrassment that you may have the first couple of times that you try something new.

Don't forget to exercise!

If you don't really know what exercises you should be doing then it may be worth thinking about going to some classes. These often cater for all fitness levels and abilities. Everyone has to start somewhere.

Once you've started exercising regularly, a good way of ensuring that you stick with it may be to find a team sport, or to sign up for a block of sessions with a particular class. The commitment to not letting the team down, or the fact that you have already paid for your class, may provide that little extra motivation (if the motivation of achieving a slim toned body isn't quite enough).

Somebody once said to me that they would have a 'celebrity' figure, if they could have a personal trainer. This maybe the case, but a personal trainer does not come around to your house and do your sit ups for you while you watch the TV. I suspect that this is another of those little excuses that often creep in when we are faced with having to take action on something important. If you honestly feel that the only way you will get fit is to have a little bit more personal supervision, then look into it. How much are you prepared to invest to be slim and healthy? Many personal trainers also run small groups, which will spread the cost, if you can find some friends to share a session with. You will still get the benefits of close supervision, even with a few of you in a group. Alternatively, it may be cheaper to get one-to-one training if you go down to the gym.

If you are looking for something a little bit different, then consider British Military Fitness (www.britmilfit.com). They run fitness sessions in local parks around the country. Each session is run by trained instructors (ex-army) and the emphasis is on improving your fitness. You will be put into groups depending on your overall fitness; however you will be encouraged to push yourself. It is perfect for you if you need a bit more of a disciplined approach to exercise, however it's not like boot camp and the instructors provide motivation, rather than shouting at you army-style! Focusing on improving fitness takes some of the pressure off losing weight. Becoming fitter will make you feel better and you will inevitably lose weight as well.

Many forms of exercise have additional benefits. Learning karate is likely to improve your self-confidence in certain situations. Yoga may help you to relax and dance classes are likely to improve your posture. You may also find that you meet people and form new social groups through exercise classes.

If you are not keen on high impact exercises then cycling, swimming and walking are all good. You can even start slowly and work your way up. It is worthwhile spending a bit of time and effort finding an exercise that will suit you.

Getting fit does not need to be expensive. It is worth investing in a good pair of trainers. Other than that, you are all good to go. Walking and running are free. Any other expenses can be seen as a good investment in your health and fitness. You don't have to be a member of an expensive gym; most run pay-per-session aerobics, circuit training and various other classes.

Swimming pools and gyms are often open from very early in the morning to quite late at night, and at weekends, giving you the flexibility to plan your exercise in at a convenient time. If you have made 'being slim' a priority for you, then you will never be too busy to fit in some exercise. Not many people, if they are being honest with themselves, can say that they cannot free up thirty minutes most days to do some exercise. Especially if they are aware that it is a good way to achieve a healthy, slim body. How often do you find yourself wasting time in front of a boring television programme? If you had given that up to do something else, you would probably not have felt like you had missed out.

Why not kill two birds with one stone and make your exercise time part of your relaxation, or social time as well? Taking the dog out for a brisk walk in the park could be a way to unwind after a day at work, or a way to prepare yourself for the day ahead, if you are a morning person. A gentle jog with a friend may be a great opportunity to catch up on the gossip, once you have got to the stage where you can run and talk at the same time.

It is crucial to enjoy exercise. Try everything until you find what you like. Any activity that you don't like, or that feels too hard, will de-motivate you. You need to enjoy this in order to stick with it, so it's important to not feel like you are punishing yourself. Ask yourself whether you enjoy this enough to continue with it in the long term. If the answer is no, then carry on only for as long as it takes you to find something that you prefer. There are lots of sports and activities out there – there is something for everyone.

For the vast majority of people, there is no good reason for not doing regular exercise, ESPECIALLY if you wish to lose weight. Attitudes towards exercise are just as prone to the justifications and excuses that often creep in to defend eating habits. If you want to lose weight and improve your health and fitness then exercise is the answer. You will see results so much quicker from introducing exercise into your new lifestyle than you would by just changing your diet on its own.

Rest and relaxation

A carefully balanced diet and regular exercise are major parts of a healthy lifestyle, but relaxation and recovery time are important too. A good nights sleep leaves you feeling refreshed whereas a bad nights sleep can ruin your day before it has even begun. If you feel less energetic due to lack of sleep it is more likely that you will go in search of a quick pick-me-up, in the form of sugar or a caffeine fix. I find that I eat more on the days when I am tired. In particular, I eat more when I have a hangover, which is probably a combination of dehydration and a lack of sleep. If you find that you need to have sugary snacks to keep you awake, then it may be worth changing your lifestyle slightly to try and fit in a bit more sleep and relaxation time. It will make you feel more energetic, so you will not need to rely on those energy fixes. Everyone is different, but for some people not getting enough sleep regularly can be a weight-gaining habit.

It's all about you

I hope that you have not reached the end of this chapter and said to yourself, "What exactly do I have to do?" This may have happened if you have been very used to dieting. Diets give you strict rules, which if you follow you will probably lose weight and if you ignore, you will probably put weight on. This is not like that. This approach is about your lifestyle, about your life. If you want to be slim, and you want to be slim for life, then you must make decisions that reflect that, MOST of the time – in the same way that slim people do. They are your choices to make. YOU must decide how to find a balance in your own life between; eating the foods that tend to cause weight gain, or deciding not to eat them; exercising regularly or choosing not to.

This is all about habits, and what you do MOST of the time. It is not about always making the 'right' choice. Whatever choices you do make, do not feel guilty about them, there is absolutely no point. Guilt makes us emotional, and we have to be rational and practical to give ourselves the best chance of becoming thin. If you happen to go on a binge, don't worry about it. Start each day afresh, prioritise being slim again and get on with it. Keep 'being slim' a priority in your life. It will help you stay focused and give you the inspiration to change your lifestyle.

Never underestimate the accumulation factor. Small things, if you do lots of them often, very quickly add up. A half an hour walk may only use up 100 calories, which may not seem worth it if you consider that it's only equivalent to a fun-sized chocolate bar. However, how hard is it to walk for half an hour? If you did it every day you would burn an extra 700 calories a week. That starts to sound a little bit more impressive. In a year that works out at 35,000 calories (with 2 weeks off). That is the equivalent of 10 lbs of fat in a year! Of course, the quicker you walk the more calories you will burn up in the same period of time.

Weight loss <u>can</u> be achieved without gym membership, and without any restrictive dieting.

'Be Slim'

When can I expect results?

One step at a time...

This is not a diet plan which starts first thing Monday, with a weigh-in and half a grapefruit for breakfast. This is your life. The rest of it!

Unlike diets, which are very restrictive, this is entirely up to you. You will still be able to eat your favourite foods; there are no restrictions, only choices. Your weight will always reflect your lifestyle; therefore it will help you to shift the focus to 'lifestyle-watching' rather than 'weight-watching'. It is up to you what you want to achieve. Bearing in mind that we cannot just wave a magic wand and make 'the weight' go away, we have two choices:

- option one is to carry on as we always have done, justifying and defending our weight, maybe giving the latest fad diet a go every now and again to see if it works for us,

- option two is deciding to change – choosing to prioritise being slim, and to alter our lifestyles in order to achieve this.

If option two sounds more appealing then congratulations, you are already on the road to becoming slim and healthy. The first stage is simple, and it is the acceptance that your lifestyle and attitudes can make a big difference to your body weight. In order to become slim, permanently, you must begin to think and act like a slim person – but this will not change who you are. You will still be the same person. The only thing that you will change about yourself is breaking the habits that were making you overweight and choosing to be slim.

Thinking like a slim person means that you accept that being slim requires a little bit of effort, and that it doesn't just come naturally. The effort is worth it of course – if you have decided that being slim is a priority for you. Remember, there is no natural advantage; even the thinnest people who overeat and fail to do sufficient exercise will put on weight. Although some effort is required to be slim and healthy, it is much less effort than going on a diet twice a year to try to undo six months worth of damage.

Not only are we constantly bombarded with pictures of thin people in the media, we are also repeatedly being told that these people don't have to work hard to stay slim. As well as sending a mixed message, it is also a big lie. No wonder 'normal' people feel like they are being cheated somehow, when they aren't able to eat whatever they please, and still be as thin as their favourite celebrity.

Look one step further, at the products which these incredibly thin celebrities are endorsing. You would be forgiven for thinking that all you have to do is buy the product and you will start to look like they do. I'm sure that the many fitness videos and 'health' foods that are being endorsed could help to make a difference, but only as part of a 'slim' lifestyle. The adverts are only providing a snapshot of a lifestyle. Take, for example, the actress who endorses a diet drink. She is not slim because of what she regularly drinks. These people are slim because they work hard at being slim. As a result of working hard at being slim, they get chosen to endorse 'slim' products to make us feel like being slim will be easy as long as we buy in to it.

A better message comes through the fitness videos, but we are still being tempted to think that we might look like a supermodel, if we did their latest workout a couple of times. All too often we buy these products, use them two or three times, and get bored. This is because doing fitness videos in our own living rooms can be dull! There is no sociable aspect to it and if we don't see results we can get disheartened and give up.

Being slim is more of a priority for these celebrities than for most people, as their livelihood very often depends upon it. I do believe that there is a pressure to remain too thin in a lot of cases! Instead of being honest and admitting that the super-toned body is a result of two hours in the gym every day, it seems to be the done thing to deny any hint of hard work. This is because people do not want to be seen to be working very hard at something that appears to come naturally to the next woman. Unfortunately, it does not come naturally to the next woman either. No wonder us mere mortals are left confused.

Have realistic expectations of 'normal', 'healthy' and 'slim'!

A normal, healthy weight is very achievable with a normal, healthy lifestyle. A super skinny body takes it to the next level, where you have to actively deprive yourself of certain foods or do a serious amount of exercise to achieve it. Maintaining it, once you are there, is also very hard work. It is highly likely that many of the very thin people, who rely on having nice figures as part of their jobs, do not indulge very often. These people probably never 'take a holiday' from being a slim person. It is their choice not to!

The pressure is immense when you consider that, as a nation, we are obsessed with photos of gorgeous celebrities looking bad for a change. Any hint of a roll of fat or a speck of cellulite gets splashed across the covers of the gossip magazines. Taking all this into account, being very thin is not to be envied. As we often see photographs of celebrities looking 'normal' in between films, or on a career break, we can see that they are no different to anyone else. When being thin becomes less of a priority, then even gorgeous celebrities will put weight on – just like the rest of us.

If you wish to be super thin then good luck – personally, I do not think it is worth the hard work or the interference to my life. However, whilst I have that attitude, I will never achieve it. I have <u>decided</u> that I would not enjoy it and therefore I have prevented myself from ever accomplishing it. We know now that if I ever did want to be very thin, I would have to accept that I have the choice to go for it, make it a priority, and accept that I would have to work at it! At the moment though I manage to have a nice balance in my lifestyle and maintain a healthy BMI of 22. To lower this figure would undoubtedly take a lot of effort. In return I would see very little, or no, benefit to my health.

However, if it were part of my job to be very slim, or it was a priority for me, then no doubt I would put in the gym hours and be very careful when selecting my meals. If the reward was a £1 million acting or modelling contract, it may all suddenly become worth the effort!

Luckily, it is possible to enjoy a healthy lifestyle and be slim, without feeling that you are on a restrictive diet, or feeling guilty that you are not spending every waking moment in the gym. It is about finding a nice balance, and having a lifestyle which you enjoy, where being slim and healthy is a priority.

Don't be fooled by the media; many celebrities work extremely hard to stay slim – it is part of their job

Hopefully, it helps to know that being very slim does not come naturally to anybody. Having a realistic goal of a healthy, slim weight is much easier to achieve than aiming to be very thin. Along with making the choice to go for it, it is also important that you decide that you will enjoy it, and work out what suits you the best. After all here, we are talking about your life. If you are determined to view any lifestyle change as restrictive, or like a diet, then unfortunately you are setting yourself up for a fall. You will sabotage your own efforts to lose weight. The more you enjoy introducing changes, and seeing the benefits of those changes, the more successful you will be in the long-run.

Enjoy it!

Deciding to enjoy weight loss may seem very alien to the regular dieter who is used to the miserable feeling of being on a diet. You are allowed to enjoy this! Concentrate on all of the freedom that comes with being able to choose. You are <u>not</u> on a diet of mung beans, or cabbage soup. You are allowed carbohydrates and protein in the same meal, and you can eat at any time of the day. YOU get to <u>choose</u> what you eat, how much you eat, and how much exercise you do. The only framework is that the more slim, healthy food choices that you make and the more that you exercise, the more remarkable the improvement in your fitness and health will be. As a consequence, the more noticeable the weight loss will be. You call the shots.

It helps to balance the enjoyment factor against impact factor. By that I mean, the impact that a particular habit has on your ultimate goal of being slim and healthy. If you really enjoy something and it is not detrimental to your health, or your waistline, then there is no reason not to carry on with it. At some point you are bound to come across something which you love doing, but it doesn't really fit in with the 'slim' priorities. That is when the priorities really get tested – when you have to make a tough decision.

It is important to enjoy being able to choose

Make sure that you judge each habit (and its priority) independently. If you change nine out of ten unhealthy habits for healthy ones, the one habit that you have kept, because it is important to you, should not seriously impede your progress. This is not an all-or-nothing approach, like diets often are. The more 'slim' choices you make, the more impressive the results will be. Try not to justify, or defend a habit, and be honest with yourself if you notice old excuses creeping back in.

Some habits you will not want to let go of easily, some not at all. That is fine; it is your choice.

Lots of small changes will add up to a big difference

A complete lifestyle overhaul would be very ambitious and probably unnecessary for most people. You do not need to leave behind the 'old' you, just make adjustments to some of the things that you do (or more importantly, don't do). The more adjustments that you make, the more impressive the results will be.

Remember that each time you decide that something is more important to you than being slim, then 'being slim' will move slightly further down your list of priorities. Do it often enough and you will be less likely to achieve slimness, as it is not a priority for you. If you do want to be slim, it must be fairly high up on your list of priorities, like it is for many slim people! You can be slim, but first you must decide that it is a priority, and keep reminding yourself that it is a priority.

Keep changing

Anything that you do not enjoy doing will very quickly become boring or irritating. That is why it is important to keep a nice balance of things that you enjoy, which will help you to cope better with the things that are not so enjoyable or exciting. One easy way to avoid getting bored is to keep changing. Try new foods, even foods that you think you may not like – you might surprise yourself. If you have decided that you are going to eat more fruit and vegetables in place of unhealthy snacks, it would quickly become very frustrating to eat the same, unexciting alternative every single day. A week of eating carrot sticks instead of chocolate bars would be enough to drive anybody back to the old habits. Be inventive, try smoothies, yoghurt, nuts, a bowl of cereal, or aim for a different fruit every day. If a chocolate bar used to be a daily habit then deciding to have an alternative most days and a fun-size bar every now and again is still a massive step in the right direction. Remember, this is not punishment, only a set of lifestyle choices which you have to be happy with.

Do what you need to do!

Whether you have tried weight-loss diets before or not, you may find this new lifestyle approach a little bit strange. In some ways dieting is easier because it does not require you to think about what you are doing, you just have to follow instructions. Admittedly, that in itself is fairly tough, when all you want is a chip butty. The frequent dieters may be the ones who will find it the hardest to let go of the guilt, the excuses, and the tendency to rebel against the diet.

It is not too important to get hung up on the exact calorie content of a particular food, or to know exactly how many grams of fat there are in your dessert. Just generalise a bit; more fruit and vegetables, less dessert; more walking, less driving; maybe a little bit less food at each meal – but still enough to feel satisfied. You can set your own rules. Maybe you don't want to give up your pub time, but could you consider swapping the kebab that inevitably follows for a bowl of cereal before bed? If you enjoy eating whilst watching a film – would it be so terrible to break that habit, if the ultimate reward was to be slim? If the answer is yes, and it is important to you to eat while watching a film, then why not consider a compromise? How about you treat yourself to popcorn at the cinema, but don't eat when watching films at home? Alternatively, find another trade-off, and walk to the cinema.

Remember, any compromise is a deal between yourself and your goal of being slim. It is not a bargain that you have made with the 'evil diet'. It is important to be able to spot if justifications and defensive behaviours start creeping in. Eat while watching a film if you <u>choose</u>

to, but not because you feel that you <u>deserve</u> to, and certainly not just because everyone else is doing it.

Noticing as many little habits as possible and taking action on some of them WILL make a difference. Where you aren't ready to change completely, try a compromise.

You deserve to be slim and healthy

Live like your life depended on it

Have you ever considered what you might do if you were told that you had to lose weight and improve your lifestyle for the sake of your health? Hopefully you will never find yourself in this position, but for some people, this is the only thing that motivates them to change their unhealthy ways. By this last-resort stage, their bodies have undoubtedly suffered decades of abuse, and unhealthy habits would be so ingrained that they would be extremely difficult to change. There is also a good chance that someone in this situation would already be suffering with an underlying medical condition which has prompted the doctor's warning.

Prioritising health and fitness now is an investment in your future

Why wait until you have been told that your cholesterol levels are too high, or that your joints, or more importantly, your heart, can't cope with your excess weight? It is possible to minimise the chances of this happening to you by taking action to avoid it now. If you make healthy lifestyle choices, then you will reap the benefits of a much healthier body in the years to come. It may sound dramatic to say that you need to *live like your life depended on it,* but it is true; how healthy you are, is often a reflection of how healthy your lifestyle is.

Even if you are not especially overweight and only want to lose a couple of excess pounds, there will still be health benefits with your new healthy lifestyle. This is especially true when you consider the accumulation factor, where a couple of pounds here and there will add up to stones eventually.

This is why it is important to prioritise being healthy, as well as slim. The pressures of modern day living often push health and fitness onto the back-burner. More immediate concerns take a higher priority, and health only becomes a priority once it is lost; being slim only becomes a priority once we have already begun to gain weight. Why wait and risk your health for the sake of other things in life? In the short term these may seem to be highly important, but, in the long term they would be meaningless if you did not have the good health to enjoy them. Investing time and effort into your health and well-being now, and permanently, will save you a huge job in the future – and you never know, it might just save your life!

Being as fit and healthy as you can be will give you more energy to enjoy the important things in life. You deserve to be as fit and healthy as you possibly can. It's just an added bonus that you will be slim as well.

Time-scales

Once you have accepted that in order to be slim your habits need to change, and start to make changes to your lifestyle, you can stop worrying about your weight. Most dieters put lots of effort into losing weight quickly, only to start putting it back on again once they are free from the diet regime. Why is there a great panic to lose weight ever so quickly?

If you were on a restrictive diet, you would want to lose weight quickly for two reasons. Firstly, the diet is making you miserable and you would want to finish it as soon as possible. Secondly, because the diet is so hard, you feel that you need to see instant results in order to justify the effort that you have gone to. Neither of those situations applies to the lifestyle approach.

By adopting the lifestyle approach to weight loss you should not be miserable, or feel like you are missing out on life. Also, it is not so much hard work that you feel you need an instant pay-off. If you spent a year living a lifestyle that you enjoyed and putting weight on, is it not reasonable to make some small changes to that lifestyle, so that you still enjoy it, but you also lose that weight over that same time period? Obviously, the more dramatically your lifestyle changes, the quicker that you will see the results that you want. Still it helps to be realistic. If you have put weight on gradually over four or five years then it is not very realistic to aim to lose all that weight in a single month. However, it may be very feasible to aim to have lost most of that weight by this time next year. Only you will know your time-scales and what your aims should be.

It might be worth taking a few minutes now to write down your targets. It might be helpful to refer to your habit lists from earlier when thinking about what your targets are going to be. Now, think of a date in the future which is a reasonable time period away; for example, your next birthday, or your friend's wedding, maybe even this day next year. Now write down all your targets. This doesn't have to include a target weight – it could be a lot more general then that – for example "I want to be losing weight", or "I want to feel in control of my weight", or, more specifically, "I want to be able to fit into a lower dress size".

Refer back to your personalised Action Plan and identify as many lifestyle habits as you think that you might need in order to achieve your target within the time frame that you have set. With your lifestyle targets it may help to be very specific such as, "I want to be in the habit of eating five portions of fruit and vegetables a day", "I want to swim 40 lengths every week", and "I want to have stopped taking sugar in hot drinks". Remember that the little things really add up.

If you want to just lose 'some' weight in the next six months, you may chose to change a few small eating habits and decide to do a bit more exercise. If you feel you need to lose three stones and want to have achieved it a year from now, then you may decide that a few big changes, in addition to many little changes are required.

Incidentally, losing three stones sounds like a major challenge, but taken slowly and surely over a long enough period of time, you can lose that weight and maintain it permanently, without feeling restricted or that you are putting your life on hold. At the rate of a pound a week, theoretically it will take less than ten months to lose three stones. However, we all know that even the best laid weight-loss plans are often not that simple. Allow time for your weight to reflect your lifestyle – concentrate more on lifestyle-watching rather than weight-watching. If you are making slow progress, review your habit list and ask yourself whether your lifestyle has changed enough? Are you still making 'being slim' a priority? If you are making good progress, analyse what you are doing to make it happen, so that you carry on moving towards your target.

Remember that this does not mean that you will spend those ten months on a diet. Think instead in terms of starting a new permanent lifestyle which you will enjoy. It just so happens that as a result you will also notice substantial weight loss.

This allows you to think carefully about your priorities and will help relieve some of the panic that can often set in when people get hung-up on rigid time-scales. It may seem daunting at first to have this big list of lifestyle changes, so maybe you want to consider changing a habit a week and really get used to one small change at a time. Planning can help you to prioritise and it is helpful to leave yourself sufficient time to start to see results.

Imagine yourself in two or three year's time. Do you want to be slim, and leading a healthy lifestyle which you enjoy? Do you want to be in a position where you no longer feel like you have to diet, or constantly worry about your weight? In two or three year's time, will it matter whether you managed to lose the weight in a month or in three months, or a year? The important thing will be that you managed to lose the weight and not put it back on. That is worth so much more than losing weight quickly. Losing excess, unhealthy weight, which stays off for the rest of your life, due to your new healthy habits, is much better done properly than quickly.

Focus on the weight you want to be for the rest of your life

Working out how long it has taken you to gain the weight can help you work out what it is about your lifestyle which may have been contributing to your excess weight. If you have been steadily gaining weight since you started to work a new shift pattern, then maybe you need to solve the problems associated with eating and sleeping at strange times, in order to begin to lose weight. Maybe a simple change in routine is all that is required to start losing weight. However, is it also possible that you have been using 'shift patterns' as an excuse, leaving you feeling like you were not in control of your choices? This example obviously does not apply to everyone. However it is worth trying to analyse your own situation as thoroughly as possible.

Some lifestyle changes which can cause weight gain are more transparent than others. For example, it is obvious that 'baby weight' is due to a pregnancy, and the time-scale was nine months. So instead of feeling tremendous pressure to bounce back into shape in a matter of weeks like many celebrities seem to do, why not aim to lose the weight over several months – nine, perhaps? Of course, it may be difficult to feel completely in control of your lifestyle after such a life-changing event, but it is important not to use 'the baby' as a false justification for excess weight later on. Blaming the 'baby weight' when the kids are old enough to be in school doesn't really work very well!

If you have not yet had children then the best advice is to not put too much 'baby weight' on in the first place. It might seem like a nice opportunity to eat whatever you please for a while, but you will have a harder job fitting back into your pre-pregnancy jeans. It is not recommended that you diet during pregnancy, but neither is there any requirement to eat for two. The additional energy requirements for a pregnant woman are approximately 300 extra calories per day. That is roughly equivalent to a banana and a glass of milk. A healthy balanced diet, with treats in moderation should be adequate for a healthy pregnancy.[5]

If you do have children, then it can be very rewarding to know that you are teaching them the good habits that will ensure that they are healthy for life. With so many overweight children facing the prospect of adult obesity diseases, it is vital that we teach our kids how to be healthy and slim.

Avoid slipping back into old habits

Keep in mind that the harder you work at your new lifestyle, the more impressive your eventual weight loss will be. There is bound to be a short time delay between starting your 'new ways' and seeing your new, slim body emerging, but keep motivated during this time by reminding yourself that it *will* happen and it *will* be permanent, as long as the slim lifestyle habits remain.

Remembering that a habit is something that you *usually* do, but not necessarily always do, means that if you relapse into an old habit for whatever reason, there is no need to feel guilty and start sabotaging the new plan. It is what you do *most* of the time which has the biggest impact on your lifestyle. Now that you are more aware that your lifestyle dictates your weight, do not dwell on small setbacks, but

5   As always, consult your doctor for more personal advice.

concentrate on the benefits of the healthier, slim habits to get you back on track.

Your new slim lifestyle will take some getting used to. Changes in attitude may happen fairly quickly, however changing habits may take more time and practice. There are bound to be times when living like a slim person goes on the backburner for a while.

It is very important not to feel like you have somehow failed if you have a day or two where 'being slim' has been pushed down the priorities list. Use any odd slips as opportunities to learn more about yourself and your slim lifestyle. You may need to spend a bit of time refocusing on your slim goals. Or you may have gone the other way and made so many drastic changes to your lifestyle that you found it difficult to maintain. If this is the case, relax and give yourself a chance to get used to the new slim thinking first and take small steps to get back on track.

Maybe you have been living like a slim person all week and then one day you get stuck in traffic on your way home from work. You haven't got a healthy snack with you (as you didn't think that you would need it) and you get so hungry that you end up buying a chocolate bar or overeating later on at dinnertime.

If something like this happens to you, don't feel guilty about it, just learn from it so in future, unexpected situations have less effect on your slim lifestyle. You have not failed at being slim. However, work out what you are going to do if that situation (which caused you to overeat) arises in the future. This may mean keeping a non-perishable snack in the car, or having a 'Plan B' such as a very quick and easy meal in reserve at home for such occasions (for example, a ready-meal, or quick-cook pasta and a jar of sauce). Plan B meals may not be the healthiest option, or the most exciting, however they allow you to feel like you are still in control of what you eat and how much you eat, which is an important part of your slim lifestyle.

Let's look at another scenario. What happens if you are quite stressed at work and have a glass of wine in the evening to relax and before you know it you have finished the bottle? You may find that 'being slim' is relatively easy most of the time, but becomes more difficult when you are stressed. Learn from it and look at how you can deal with the stress whilst keeping 'being slim' a priority.

It may be that you need to change a small habit and pour yourself a glass of wine and then take the bottle back into the kitchen and put the cork back in. When you have finished you then have to consciously decide to get up and get another glass rather than not notice automatically pouring one. It is totally up to you to choose how many glasses you have, but the important thing is that you have <u>chosen</u> rather than just consumed without realising.

Steven

Steven read "Thin Secrets" and wanted to see for himself whether he could lose weight by thinking and acting like a slim person. For the first few days "The Secrets" were very fresh in his mind and 'being slim' was a priority for him. He made 'slim' food choices all week, including the dinner that he ordered in a restaurant. Not only was he beginning to look at his whole lifestyle, but he also started to notice how other peoples' habits were helping to keep them slim.

Steven would often go for long walks in the countryside at the weekends and he would usually have a big, relatively unhealthy lunch before he set off. On this particular Saturday, Steven was feeling so enthusiastic about 'being slim', that he opted to only have a bowl of soup and a slice of bread for his lunch. Surprisingly he felt satisfied after the small meal and went out for his usual walk armed with his healthy snack (banana) just in case.

Unfortunately for Steven it was not long before he was really quite hungry and his snack did not satisfy. When he got home, Steven had a cup of tea and some biscuits and before he knew it he had eaten half the packet. He then felt guilty and thought that he wasn't very good at 'being slim'. It took a while for Steven to realise that he had not failed at being slim but that he was still learning the best ways to change his lifestyle. He realised that he probably should have had a large lunch before walking. If this was a healthier lunch than usual then he was still making progress at 'being slim'. Alternatively, he could have had a small lunch and taken a sandwich with him.

Steven's example highlights one of the major differences between a healthy lifestyle and the diet culture. A diet would have encouraged the very small lunch and then relied on Steven's own willpower to prevent him from eating the biscuits when he got home. With a healthy lifestyle it is all about having a nice balance, which will still result in weight loss. It is uncomfortable and not particularly good for anyone to eat less than they need on the days that they are exercising. However, filling up on healthy food rather than high-calorie food means that you can still always feel full after a meal and you are much more likely to lose weight. Being slim is not about being hungry.

Be aware that being too focused on being slim very quickly may actually slow you down in the long run. It is easy to plan a very strict regime for yourself at the start of the week when you are not hungry, or stressed, or busy; but how will you feel if you don't achieve everything you set out to? Whatever the circumstances, if you do something which does not fit in with your new slim approach, do not feel guilty and do not feel like you have failed. You can be slim and there will be times where it is not very easy, but take each day as it comes, choose to be slim and prioritise being slim. The better you are at thinking and acting like a slim person, the easier it will become for you.

Keep track

This is a matter of personal choice, but as well as planning your goals, you may find it useful to monitor your progress. This can be in the form of a weekly weight chart, or a daily food or exercise diary. I personally recommend not using weight as your only measure of progress, but notice changes to the way that your clothes feel, and maybe even keep a log of your vital statistics. If you just focus on your weight then it is very easy to give up if the scales aren't telling you what you want them too. Don't give up, your weight will reflect your lifestyle, but it may take a while to get there! It might also be useful to keep a note of the 'bad' habits that you identify for change. At times where you feel that you are not making very much progress, you can look back at how the 'old you' behaved and be able to see how far you have come on the road to achieving a slim, healthy body.

If you keep track along the way, it will also be much easier to spot the changes. This means you will start to notice yourself slipping back into old habits and be able to take action. More importantly it may give you more of an idea of what works best for you. Noticing an inch off the waist, a month after introducing daily sit-ups, for example, would allow you to see the link between what you do and the results that you get. I know that if I could see a link like that I would be more motivated to do sit-ups in the future!

The best ways to develop and maintain new habits are to see the benefits of those habits. Unlike a diet programme, where the only measure of success is your weight, changing to a slim, healthier lifestyle will have a whole host of other benefits. In particular, take notice of any changes in your mood, or sleep patterns, or in your general sense of well-being and self-esteem. You may find that you get an enormous amount of satisfaction from taking control over an area of your life which you used to feel had control over you. Notice how your body changes as you increase your levels of activity. If you used to get out of breath reaching for the TV remote, observe how your fitness levels improve very quickly with regular exercise. If you choose to take up walking or jogging with a friend, then see the benefits that this will also have on your relationship.

Get some 'slim' support

Have you ever discussed dieting and weight loss with someone who is in exactly the same position as you are? This is perfectly natural, we like to talk to people about things that we have in common. Now think, have you actually discussed weight loss with a slim person? This is less likely for many reasons. Maybe we assume that our slim friends will not be sympathetic; maybe they will not understand as they can't possibly have the same problems can they? Maybe, deep down we think that our slim friends might be judging us because of our weight. Whatever your worries may be, I am sure that real friends will not judge and they will do their best to understand and help you with something that means a lot to you.

Your slim friends are probably the best source of support for your new lifestyle; after all, you will be thinking and acting like them from now on so why not learn all you can from them? They may well feel flattered that you admire their lifestyles and acknowledge the effort that they go to, and I bet that they would be very happy to help you out.

If you were a tourist and were lost, you would probably look for someone who knew where they were, so you could ask for directions. It would not make much sense to ask another lost tourist to help you find your way. Why not then ask a slim person for advice if you want to become slim? There is a bit of logic to that.

Slim people are not 'on the other side'; you should not feel like they are the competition. You may find someone who appreciates the compliment that you pay them by admitting that they do a good job of keeping themselves slim. By understanding that people are slim by choice and not begrudging them for their 'better luck', you are much more likely to get a favourable response if you ask for advice.

Find some 'slim' support

If people do not encourage you in your pursuit of a slimmer, healthier lifestyle, then do not discuss it with them. Although it is always nice to have support, you *can* do this on your own.

Finding a friend who is also trying to lose weight, and helping each other develop and maintain new habits, may help keep you focused.

However, make sure that they are also committed; you do not want them falling off the wagon and taking you with them. If you approach a friend who is reluctant to accept that they must change their attitudes and lifestyle in order to lose weight, then do not argue with them and leave them to their own devices. When they begin to notice the positive changes in you, they will become convinced.

Don't let anybody or anything hold you back from this – it is your opportunity to regain control of your weight. There are many people who do not like change as it scares them. As well as not wanting change for themselves, they can also be reluctant to accept that others around them change. If the people close to you do not react very well to your new lifestyle don't be disheartened. Explain to them that;

You are NOT changing <u>who</u> you are, only what you do

This is your life and you should feel as though you are in control. It is up to you to do as little or as much as you want to introduce slim and healthy habits.

A good motivator is reward. Try and find a way of not relying on 'nice' food for treats; focusing on the ultimate reward of a slim body should help with that, although we all get a boost from short term rewards as well. Treating yourself, and living like a slim person, need not conflict, although the treat habit may need to change. Why not visit a friend, go to the cinema, or go bowling, take a bubble bath, have a massage, go shopping (or just window shopping) where you would usually have a food treat?

I strongly recommend that you treat yourself to new clothes when you begin to lose weight. This will have two benefits. Firstly, you will feel slimmer and more confident wearing clothes that are not baggy and which fit you properly. Secondly, having clothes that fit helps you to notice any changes more easily, which is an added boost if the weight keeps coming off; however it also allows you to notice any weight gain and you will be able to react more quickly to the changes.

From a self-esteem point of view, it is important that you do not wait until you have lost a lot of weight before you buy new clothes, as you may then feel like you are putting your life on hold until you are slim. This will only lead to frustration, especially if you are not seeing fast results. The weight loss <u>will</u> happen, but you may as well look and feel your best in the meantime.

I wouldn't advise deliberately buying clothes which are too small as an incentive to stay on track, as you can't predict what shape you will be when you do lose the weight. Only buy clothes that fit and suit you and don't be scared to show off your achievements. This will really improve your confidence and help you to keep motivated by reminding you of your progress. Celebrate every couple of pounds lost (but not with food!), they all add up. Whether or not you decide to keep your old clothes (that are too big) is your choice. Personally, I believe that donating them to a charity shop would be a nice gesture; after all, you'll not need them again, will you?

Another big motivator is the knowledge that you will never again have to diet. A 'slim', healthy lifestyle will help you to lose weight and remain slim for as long as it is a priority for you. Have you ever made a New Year's resolution, to lose weight by dieting, and found it so difficult that you have given up by January 3rd? Introducing changes to both your diet and your activity levels and making those changes habit, will enable you to avoid those January resolutions. Not only that, but maintaining a constant, healthy weight means not having to diet before holidays or special occasions where you previously felt the pressure to lose a few pounds.

No more diets!

You will be able to maintain your new healthy weight by keeping an eye on the small changes and taking immediate action when old habits start to creep back in. There will be occasional overindulgences, but as these will be compensated for, they will not cause a problem in the long run. Acting on small changes early will avoid any significant weight gain and therefore ensure that the New Year diet is definitely a thing of the past.

Absolutely, the most important thing of all is that you must enjoy doing this. There will be times when it will be really tempting to revert to old habits; especially if you haven't seen immediate results (be patient, your weight <u>will</u> eventually change to reflect your lifestyle). Remember that you could sabotage this for yourself by 'deciding' that you are not going to enjoy it. Nobody is forcing you to do anything, if you do not want to become slim and healthy, then choose not to. If you decide that you do want to do this, then make sure that you enjoy the ride; it's up to you how fast you go, and in what direction.

The advantage to changing your lifestyle rather than going on a diet is that you are really investing in yourself. You are not temporarily abusing yourself in order to lose weight like you might be on a fad diet. Do not look upon this as a permanent diet – it is not. You can choose what it is that you eat and drink and how much exercise that you do (or don't do). All you have to remember is that you will only get out what you put in. It is what you do, <u>most</u> of the time that will have the biggest impact on your weight. So yes, you can choose whether or not to eat chocolate cake, knowing that you are in control over that choice, and not feeling guilty, whatever decision you make. You are aware that chocolate cake is not a 'bad' food, it is not the enemy. However you also know that if eating chocolate cake became a habit this would undoubtedly have an effect on your weight.

If you are not enjoying major lifestyle changes then go slower; just be prepared for the results to take a little longer.

What are you waiting for? Go for it!

I believe that anybody can lose weight and achieve a healthier lifestyle without obsessive calorie-counting or restrictive dieting. Keep in mind the 'big secret' – that slim people were not born with a natural advantage. Instead they are aware that being slim is a lifestyle choice and that it is the decisions and actions that you take MOST of the time that have the biggest impact on your weight. Notice the small weight changes, and the little things that you do, as these will all add up over time. If you want to be slim, you need to <u>choose</u> to be slim, <u>prioritise</u> it, and make it happen for you. You can be slim and in control of your weight.

Thinking and acting like a slim person is the key to becoming a healthy weight, which you will be able to maintain permanently. If your attitudes have changed whilst reading this book then you are already well on the way to becoming a slim person. I wish you the best of luck and I hope you enjoy it.

Develop your slim, healthy habits and weight loss <u>will</u> follow

Appendix

Calculate your body mass index

To calculate your own body mass index you will need to know your height in metres and your weight in kg (or use the conversions shown).

$$BMI = \frac{weight\ (kg)}{height\ (m^2)}$$

To convert your total weight in pounds into kilograms, divide by 2.2. To convert inches into centimetres multiply by 2.5. You will then need to divide by 100 to get your height in metres.

You can also calculate your BMI on our website www.thinsecrets.com

What is a healthy weight for your height?

	← Healthy weight range (imperial) →					
	BMI = 20		BMI = 22.5		BMI = 25	
Height	Stones	lbs	Stones	lbs	Stones	lbs
4' 10"	6	9	7	6	8	4
4' 11"	6	12	7	10	8	8
5' 0"	7	1	7	13	8	12
5' 1"	7	4	8	3	9	2
5' 2"	7	8	8	7	9	6
5' 3"	7	11	8	11	9	10
5' 4"	8	1	9	1	10	1
5' 5"	8	4	9	5	10	5
5' 6"	8	8	9	9	10	10
5' 7"	8	11	9	13	11	0
5' 8"	9	1	10	3	11	5
5' 9"	9	5	10	7	11	10
5' 10"	9	9	10	12	12	0
5' 11"	9	13	11	2	12	5
6' 0"	10	3	11	6	12	10
6' 1"	10	7	11	11	13	1
6' 2"	10	11	12	1	13	6
6' 3"	11	1	12	6	13	11

	← Healthy weight range (metric) →		
	BMI = 20	BMI = 22.5	BMI = 25
Height (cm)	kg	kg	kg
146	42.6	48.0	53.3
148	43.8	49.3	54.8
150	45.0	50.6	56.3
152	46.2	52.0	57.8
154	47.4	53.4	59.3
156	48.7	54.8	60.8
158	49.9	56.2	62.4
160	51.2	57.6	64.0
162	52.5	59.0	65.6
164	53.8	60.5	67.2
166	55.1	62.0	68.9
168	56.4	63.5	70.6
170	57.8	65.0	72.3
172	59.2	66.6	74.0
174	60.6	68.1	75.7
176	62.0	69.7	77.4
178	63.4	71.3	79.2
180	64.8	72.9	81.0
182	66.2	74.5	82.8
184	67.7	76.2	84.6
186	69.2	77.8	86.5
188	70.7	79.5	88.4

Notes

Notes

Notes